AF723335

Sirtfood Diet Cookbook

Quick and Healthy Recipes to Lose Weight. Start to Burn Fat Boosting Your Metabolism and Activating Your "Skinny Gene".

Elizabeth Baker

ISBN: 978-1-914358-88-3

Table of content

Introduction

Aidan Goggins & Glen Matten, celebrity nutritionists, developed the Sirtfood Diet in 2016. The diet, which includes foods that activate the body's skinny gene, is designed to help people lose weight quickly and without the side effects that come from most diets. Some diets necessitate starvation, which results in muscle loss as well as fat loss. Some might require you to give up foods you enjoy, rendering them so restricting that most people find it impossible to continue to them.

The Sirtfood Diet, on the other hand, enables you to consume sirtuin-rich foods that are mixed into tasty and nutritious meals for both body and mind, making it really healthy and efficient. The sirtfood diet is named after sirtuin activators, a molecule found in certain plant-based foods. Sirtuin activators are a form of protein that protects cells from the effects of aging, inflammation, and a variety of other harmful metabolic processes.

As a result, sirtuin activators are being linked to longevity, with individuals who consume large quantities of sirtuin over extended periods of time surviving much longer than their peer group. There are numerous other advantages, such as improved muscle mass as well as easier fat burning. The Sirt-food diet focuses on maintaining a strong sirtuin intake while losing weight and improving overall wellbeing. The shift in focus of the sirtfood diet is fascinating. This isn't a weight-loss fad diet;

however, the focus is on eating a nutritious, balanced diet, with weight reduction occurring gradually after your body has been purified of your bad eating habits.

Sirtuin activators can be present in a number of foods, including chocolate & red wine. Of course, the sirtuin diet does not imply to be a magical diet that allows you to eat all the sweets and drink all the wine you want. You'll also need to hold the calorie consumption in order and follow a healthy diet that contains a range of essential food groups. Apples, citrus fruits, strawberries, green tea, soy, tomatoes, turmeric, olive oil, red onion, and kale are among the balanced sirtuin activator foods used in the diet. There are a few surprises, like coffee, which is commonly despised upon in most western diets.

The Sirtfood Diet is focused on calorie restriction and the intake of a small number of foods. If you plan to follow the diet, you'll find that it's split up into two stages that last a total of 21 days—the first is seven days long, and the second is 14 days long. You can ingest just 1,000 calories a day over the first three days, which involves one meal as well as 3 Sirtfood green juices. The maximum calorie consumption is raised to 1,500 on days four and seven, and you're recommended to drink two green juices and eat two meals a day. The second phase of the diet includes 3 Sirtfood meals as well as a green juice every day. There is no calorie limit for the first 21 days, although you are advised to consume three meals rich in sirtfoods and a green juice each day if you wish to continue.

Anyone may adopt the sirtfood diet; it is not pricey, time-consuming, or hard to prepare. It does, though, necessitate the use of a juicer, which you would need to buy if you do not already have one. Also, with lower intensities or no activity, the body can let go of excess fat with a slight calorie restriction and a rise in sirtuin-rich foods.

Matten and Goggins proved that the overwhelming majority of participants lost a considerable amount of weight, on average 7 pounds, in studies conducted prior to the diet's release. It's not all about losing weight, however. The Sirtfood Diet has been shown to boost mental and physical wellbeing. Overall, there are some compelling reasons to start thinking about the Sirtfood Diet—if you want to lose weight, build muscle, and improve your fitness, this is an excellent way to do so. It can take time and effort, so if you stay with it, you will enjoy these rewards as well. You will start being a healthier person on the inside and out.

Chapter 1: Understanding to Sirtfood Diet

When a celebrity sheds weight, the diet they credit for it goes viral. **Adele, the British singer,** is claimed to have adopted the "sirtfood" diet.

It entails consuming foods that increase sirtuin levels, such as blueberries, strawberries, walnuts, green tea, and also red wine & dark chocolate, along with onions and garlic.

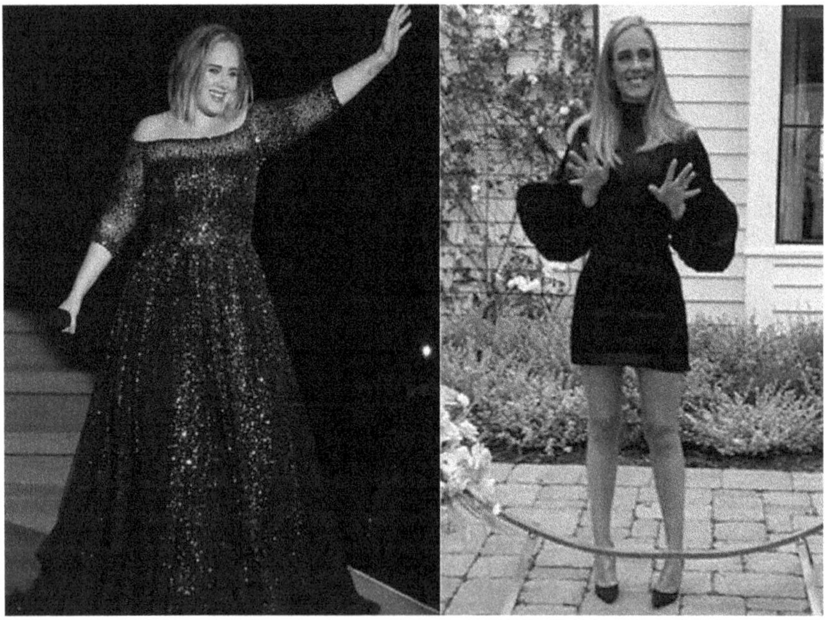

Because of inflammation-reducing compounds such as polyphenols, there's strong proof that these ingredients are nutritious and may even help you live longer.

1.1 What Is Sirtfood Diet?

Dietitians Aidan Goggins & Glen Matten developed the Sirtfood Diet in 2016. Celebrities such as Adele, Pippa Middleton, as well as former professional boxer David Haye have helped it achieve success.

It's known as a weight-loss remedy that works to help people lose 7 pounds in 7 days. Another distinctive feature of the diet is that it includes more pretentious foods such as dark chocolate & red wine alongside conventional, nutritious options such as kale, strawberries, as well as other whole foods.

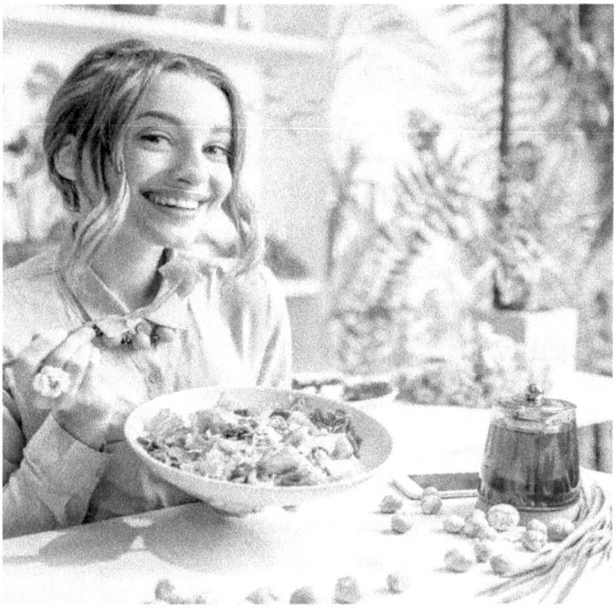

While the plan claims to put dieters on a fast track to losing weight, it still promotes severe calorie restriction. The Sirtfood Diet is focused on polyphenols, which are natural compounds present in fruits and vegetables.

According to Goggins and Matten, certain polyphenols imitate the symptoms of fasting and workout by stimulating sirtuin proteins in the body.

Sirtuins, also called SIRTs or silent information regulators, perform a role in how the body metabolizes sugar & retains fat, especially during fasting or intense caloric restriction. They could be useful in the treatment of obesity, according to a 2016 report posted in the International Journal of Molecular Sciences. Even so, the evidence is still in its inception, and the majority of the study is based on animals or human cells instead of human testing.

To stimulate sirtuins in the body, Goggins and Matten suggest consuming a number of polyphenol-rich foods as part of the Sirtfood Diet. These foods are known as "sirtfoods," hence the diet's name. However, scientists are also researching how polyphenols influence sirtuins in the body and whether they can help people lose weight.

While the recommended foods could stimulate sirtuins, this does not indicate that you can shed pounds purely as a result of them. You lose the weight primarily as a result of caloric restriction at first, as well as eating 'reasonably' balanced."

1.2 Theory of Sirtfood Diet

According to dietician Sophie, "the theory behind The Sirtfood Diet is that there are several foods that we can consume that maximize our development of a group of proteins named sirtuins." "Sirtuins are believed to serve a variety of tasks, including assisting our bodies in being more energy productive in low-calorie conditions, including dieting. The diet seems to be based around the premise that if you consume foods that assist in the production of more sirtuins, you will burn fat more quickly, and the metabolic rate will increase."

According to the authors of the Sirtfood Diet, it's a way to lose weight without being on a fad diet because it stimulates the same'skinny gene' mechanisms as fasting or exercise does. "Polyphenols are chemicals found in some foods that cause moderate stress in our bodies, activating genes that imitate the symptoms of fasting and exercise. Polyphenol-rich foods, such as kale, dark chocolate, and red wine, activate sirtuin pathways, which affect metabolism, aging, and mood. A diet abundant in these superfoods jump-starts weight reduction without losing muscle mass, all while keeping the fitness in tip-top health, "they claim.

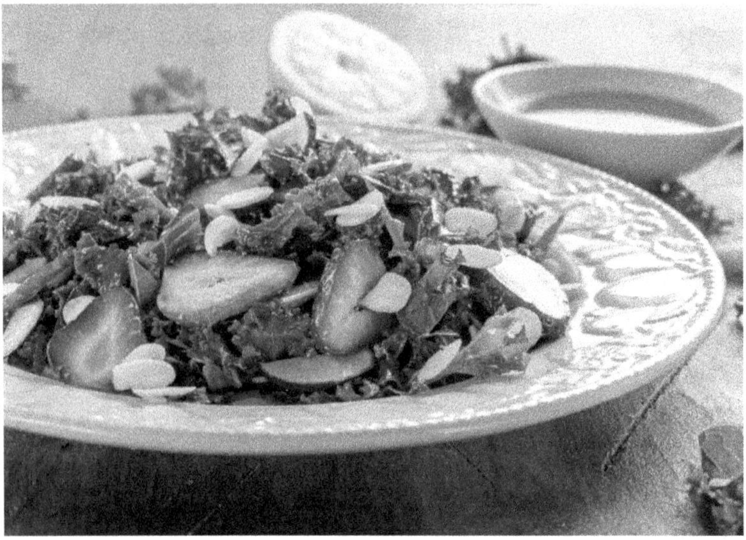

There are findings to support the belief that foods like chili and green tea will help you lose weight, and red wine (which is high in polyphenols) is often quoted as a key component in the French Paradox, which explains why French people drink red wine but remain thin. However, there is no empirical proof to support the sirtfood hypothesis at this time. There is some evidence that sirtuins can have an anti-aging effect in the lab, although these trials have only been done on rats, human stem cells, and mice, not on actual humans.

1.3 What Are Sirtuins?

Sirtuins are a collection of seven proteins involved in the removal of acetyl groups from molecules. Acetyl groups adhere to DNA at various points in the nucleus of the cell, identifying and setting up the DNA for processing. Consider them a chemical post-it note that indicates what has to be transposed into a protein or enzymes for the cell to function.

Sirtuins eliminate the acetyl group at precisely the right moment, enabling the DNA to compress and shield itself from harm. Sirtuins are effectively switching a protein off. This is a necessary mechanism for the regulation of proteins involved in aging, circadian rhythm, metabolism, and cell development.

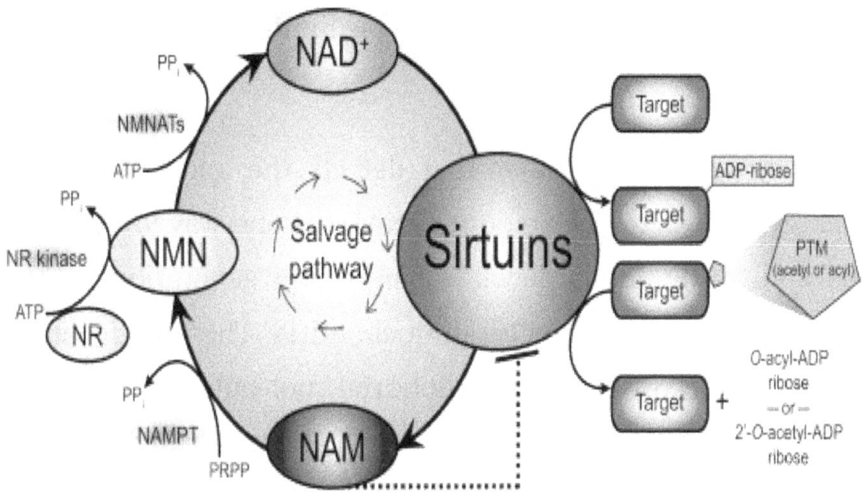

Sirtuins react to variations in a cell's energy level. Dependent on the amount of energy available, they govern the transcription of other proteins.

Most sirtuins are activated in the mitochondria and cytoplasm of the cell, in addition to replacing acetyl groups in the nucleus. These mitochondrial sirtuins play a role in the production of energy, metabolism, and cell health.

SIRT1: Energy sensor, metabolism, adipose tissue

SIRT1 is a protein found in all cells. Its role in the cell nucleus is to eliminate the acetyl groups that signify which genes can be converted into proteins. As a result, SIRT1 has an effect on whether the cell produces other proteins. It's a regulator that responds to the amount of energy in the cell.

SIRT1 is one way that certain proteins are switched off to save cellular energy while cellular energy is limited.

SIRT1 and Metabolism

SIRT1 is a cellular sensor that detects the amount of food (energy) required. The amount of NAD+ is one-way SIRT one is powered at the cellular level. During energy generation, NAD+ is generated and used in the mitochondria. The proportion of NAD+ to certain other mitochondrial molecules increases as energy is limited, such as through calorie restriction or strenuous exercise. SIRT1 expression rises in reaction to an increase in NAD+.

SIRT1 influences both average metabolic rate (and weight) as well as lifespan by influencing the expression of various proteins convoluted in metabolism, circadian rhythm, and autophagy.

SIRT1 levels fall as a result of insulin resistance. Increased SIRT1 levels have been shown to increase insulin sensitivity, particularly in cases of insulin resistance. SIRT1 achieves this by inhibiting the translation of PTP1B, a protein tyrosine phosphatase that controls insulin signaling.

SIRT1 is increased by calorie restriction (consuming 40% fewer calories than usual). It's believed to be a process by which calorie restriction improves animal lifespan.

SIRT1 in fat cells: Adipose tissue (fat cells) may be white or brown in color.

White adipose tissue, or fat, can be seen all over the body (for example, the belly, love handles, legs, and so on).

Brown adipose tissue, also known as brown fat, is a healthy kind of fat that consumes a ton of calories. It holds babies warm by generating heat without causing them to shiver.

SIRT1 activates PPAR, causing brown adipose tissue to develop and white adipose tissue to form.

SIRT1 and cancer: When we get older, it's crucial to remember to find a compromise between the need for cellular regeneration and the protection of cancerous cells growing out of control.

Although it might seem that the SIRT1 is often a good idea, there may be trade-offs whenever it comes to stopping cancerous cells from being damaged.

SIRT1 regulates the autophagy gene p53, which is essential for autophagy. This is a tumor suppressor gene that has to be present in the appropriate number of cells in order to enable cancerous cell death. The p53 protein inhibits cell division, allowing for either DNA repair or apoptosis (cell death).

Inhibiting SIRT1 has been shown to help combat cancer in a variety of animal and cell studies.

SIRT3: Metabolism and Longevity

SIRT3 is a mitochondrial protein that has been researched for its function in aging and metabolic syndrome. It regulates the expression of many essential mitochondrial genes. Longevity is linked to higher amounts of SIRT3.

SIRT3 & Metabolism

SIRT3 is also essential in metabolism, and mice lacking SIRT3 on a high-fat diet had more obesity and insulin resistance. SIRT3 activity reduction has been related to mitochondrial impairment and metabolic syndrome.

SIRT3 influences the action of proteins necessary for mitochondrial function, such as those involved in fatty acid oxidation and oxidative stress reduction. Researchers discovered that both cold exposure and calorie restriction up-regulate SIRT3.

The role of SIRT3 is also essential in cancer prevention. Human breast cancer tissue displays SIRT3 deletion in 40% of carcinomas, and mice with the gene removed are more likely to produce tumors.

Noise-induced hearing loss in mice may be avoided with nicotinamide riboside, a counterpart to NAD+ (nicotinamide adenine dinucleotide) and a vitamin B3 derivative, according to a report published in Cell Metabolism in December 2014. In the mitochondria, the researchers discovered that nicotinamide riboside enabled SIRT3. Noise-induced hearing deterioration was avoided by increasing SIRT3. Furthermore, nicotinamide riboside (NR) supplementation was useful before and after hearing loss.

Other research suggests that calorie restriction decreases age-related hearing loss by increasing SIRT3 and "promoting the glutathione-mediated mitochondrial antioxidant protection system."

SIRT1 binds to SIRT3 and modifies it post-transnationally.

SIRT1 deacetylates SIRT3 in a post-translational way. Acetyl groups may also affect proteins after they've been produced, and acetylation and deacetylation of a protein can alter its role in a cell.

The SIRT1 protein can control SIRT3 behavior and mitochondrial function in the case of SIRT3.

We often imagine modifying a single gene to change a single function, as though we were turning a knob to switch something on or off. However, it's always more complex than just that particular lever; sirtuin interactions can often play a role in general metabolism.

Mitochondrial energy, gluconeogenesis, as well as cancer prevention are all linked to SIRT6.

- SIRT6 is also active in the processing of mitochondrial energy.
- SIRT6 assists in the regulation of glucose content in the liver while fasting. The liver processes glucose to control blood glucose levels, a process known as gluconeogenesis. SIRT6 operates with a variety of other proteins to switch on and off genes that govern the development of glucose in the liver. SIRT6 amounts are lowered in animal models of obesity and diabetes.
- SIRT6 often detects a kind of DNA damage known as double-strand splits, which is harmful to a cell. SIRT6 stimulates the DNA damage response, which helps to restore chromosome damage.

Sirtuins and NAD+

When the cell is stressed, the proportion of NAD+ to NADH changes. Lack of food (calorie reduction for a few days), strenuous exercise, and oxidative stress are all examples of this. Sirtuins function as tension adaptors by detecting variations in NAD+ levels.

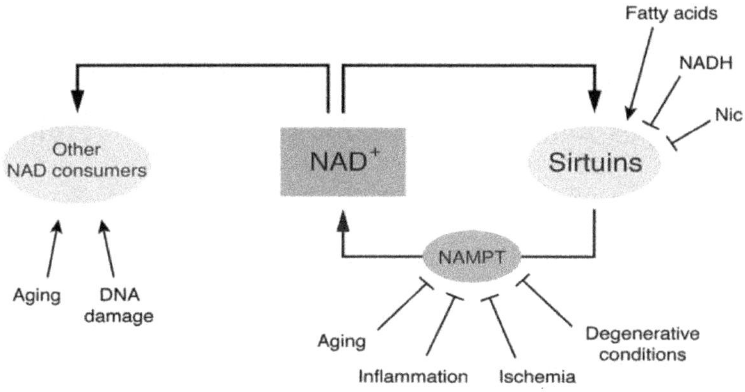

Alternatively, supplements like nicotinamide riboside (NR) will boost NAD+ levels, causing the NAD+ to NADH ratio to change in favor of SIRT1 and SIRT3 expression.

Supplements to boost sirtuins

Although foods in the diet may or may not enhance sirtuin activity at the dietary stagc, clinical studies have shown that the accompanying plant compounds influence sirtuins at levels done by taking supplements.

Resveratrol:

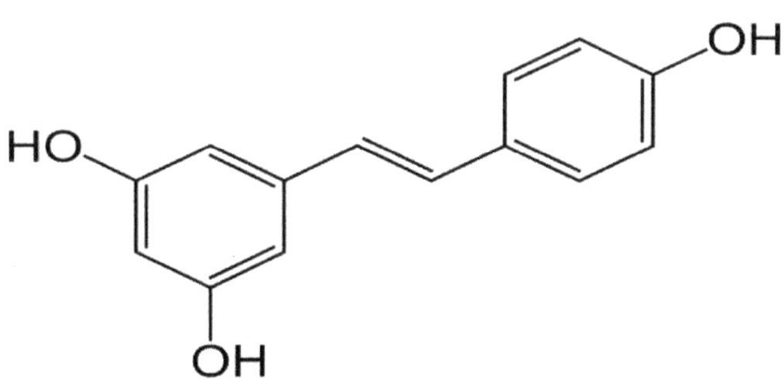

Resveratrol has been shown to work on SIRT1 in a way that inhibits AMPK, which promotes energy usage and enhances metabolism at higher doses. About 2 mg of resveratrol can be present in a bottle of red wine. Dietary consumption from foods like red grapes, almonds, and peanuts is less than one milligram a day.

Resveratrol supplement doses vary from 150 mg to 1,000 mg. This will be the equivalent of a large quantity of wine (75 glasses and up per day).

- In a limited clinical study of older adults, 1,000 mg of resveratrol administered every day for four weeks lowered post-prandial glucose reaction.
- The usage of 2,000 mg of resveratrol a day in a clinical study had almost no effect on insulin sensitivity, but Caucasians in the trials had increased insulin resistance.
- Another research showed that taking 150 mg of resveratrol would have little effect on insulin resistance.

Curcumin:

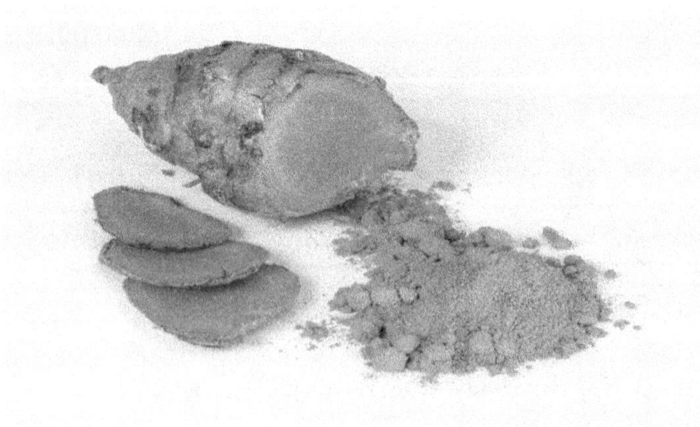

Turmeric contains a polyphenol called curcumin. Supplemental amounts of curcumin have been shown to raise SIRT1 levels in studies.

Quercetin:

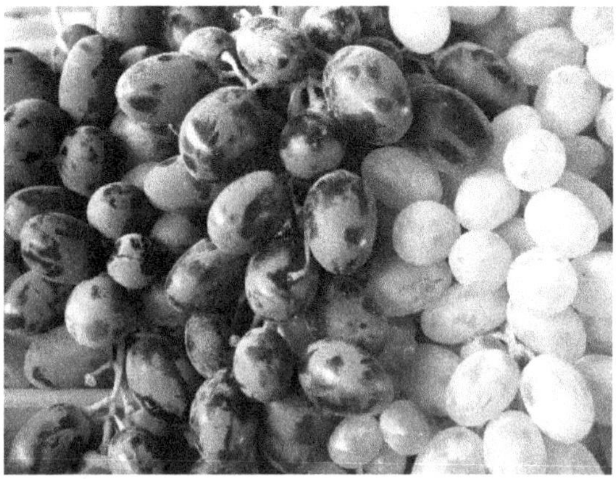

Onion, dock (sorrel), apples, watercress, elderberry, and red grapes all contain quercetin, a polyphenol. Supplemental quercetin has been shown to improve SIRT1 behavior in experiments.

Berberine:

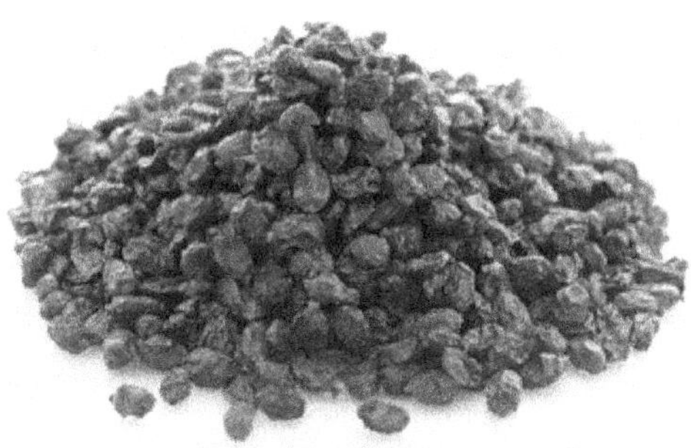

Berberine is a plant product that has been used for decades in Chinese medicine. It has been shown in studies to improve SIRT1 expression.

Nicotinamide Riboside (NR):

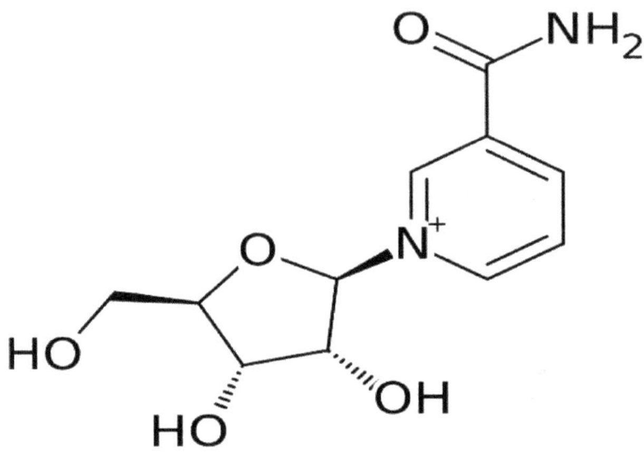

NAD+ amounts may be increased by taking a supplement called nicotinamide riboside (NR). SIRT1, as well as SIRT3 expression, are improved as the proportion of NAD+ to NADH is increased.

Vitamin D, Resveratrol, and SIRT1:

SIRT1 has an interesting interaction with vitamin D.

Vitamin D is acquired by supplementation or sun exposure. The molecule must be transformed into an active type of vitamin D (1, 25 D) and then function on a vitamin D receptor in any case. The active type of vitamin D interacting with a vitamin D receptor is essential for bone health, cell oxidative stress reduction, immune system control, and heart health, among other items. The active source of vitamin D achieves a great deal, but only because it works in tandem with the vitamin D receptor.

According to studies, increasing SIRT1 activity with resveratrol induces an improvement in vitamin D receptors. This change, when combined with the active form of vitamin D, boosts vitamin D's beneficial impact on a variety of body systems.

Drugs that bind with sirtuins contain the following:

The other half of the issue is that you want to be sure that a drug you're taking isn't sabotaging your efforts to increase sirtuins.

- Statins, which are used to reduce cholesterol, have been found to inhibit SIRT6 specifically.
- The most commonly consumed drug, alcohol, reduced SIRT1 activity in the liver.
- SIRT1 has been shown to be inhibited by NSAIDs in several studies.
- On the other side, metformin boosts SIRT1 activity.

Final thoughts

Up-regulating the sirtuins may benefit metabolism as well as healthy aging; for someone who consumes a diet of about 2,000 calories per day, the initial step of the SIRTfood diet can up-regulate SIRT1 solely by calorie reduction.

A diet plan from either book may provide certain people with the inspiration they need to make healthier eating adjustments.

All in all, you're unlikely to get sufficiently polyphenols from the diet, like resveratrol, to stimulate the sirtuins in a significant way. Supplements will almost definitely be needed. However, the calorie reduction and whole grains included in the diet could be adequate to help you lose weight on your own.

1.4 What Is A Skinny Gene?

Many people struggle to lose weight, and others strive to gain weight. Now, a group of scientists believes they've figured out that certain people stay thin even though they eat everything they want.

The discovery may assist studies into how genes might support the battle against obesity, which really is a global health issue. The World Health Organization (WHO) estimated that 1.9 billion people aged 18 and up were overweight in 2016. About 650 million of them were overweight.

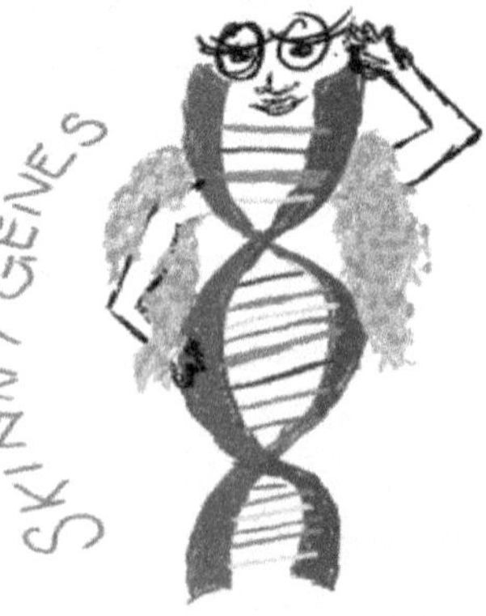

"We've all seen people: they make up only 1% of the world. They can consume anything they want and yet have a balanced metabolism. They eat a lot of food and don't often perform squats, but they don't gain weight, "According to Josef Penninger, head of the Life Sciences Department and professor in the University of British Columbia's department of medical genetics.

The **'skinny' gene** is a gene that enables individuals to be thin.

The ALK (anaplastic lymphoma kinase) gene is the variable that helps people avoid weight gain regardless of their diet. It aids in the maintenance of weight loss in thin individuals, hopefully paving the way for new obesity treatments.

In metabolically stable, thin people, the gene can play a role in preventing weight gain. It's located in the hypothalamus, which is the portion of the brain that governs appetite and fat storage.

Anaplastic lymphoma kinase is a protein generated by the ALK gene that is involved in cell development. The gene has also been related to some cancers and has been known as a tumor growth catalyst.

Variability in ALK

The researchers examined the DNA of over 47,000 individuals between the ages of 20 and 44. They examined details from Estonia's biobank, a genomic archive containing information from a significant portion of the Estonian community.

In the lower 6th percent of weight, the researchers found thin, balanced people. Those in the 30th as well as 50th percentiles, on the other side, formed the control category. Obese people were described as those in the 95th percentile. The researchers discovered gene variants that tended to be more common in slim people.

The team discovered that certain variants in the ALK gene are linked to low sensitivity to weight gain in genetically thin people after examining the database. The researchers have discovered that removing the gene resulted in thinner flies. Furthermore, mice with the ALK gene knocked out displayed marked resistance to obesity.

Treatments that target the gene

Therapeutics targeting the gene, according to the researchers, may help scientists battle obesity in the future. At the very least, people can stay thin whether the ALK gene can be turned off or its activity reduced. ALK inhibitors and other ALK therapies are widely being utilized in cancer therapy.

Before drug inhibitors are studied in humans, further testing is required to see whether they are successful for this reason. The researchers are optimistic about the study's second step, which would relate the results to biobank information on the wellbeing, DNA, and metabolic rate of other communities around the world.

The researchers also want to look at how neurons that transmit the ALK regulate metabolism and facilitate thinness in the brain at a molecular level.

Obesity and the consequences

Obesity is characterized as a body mass index (BMI) of 30 or higher in an adult. The BMI of a stable individual should be between 18.5 and 24.9. Overweight is described as a BMI greater than 25. Obesity has been linked to a number of health issues, some of which may be fatal. Type 2 diabetes, hypertension, some tumors, stroke, respiratory failure, elevated cholesterol, gallbladder disease, including fatty liver disease, are only a few of them.

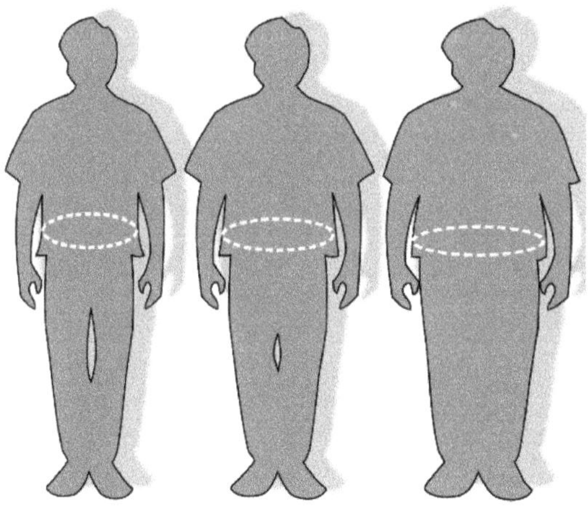

Obese patients are often more prone to have osteoarthritis, sleep apnea, and respiratory issues, as well as psychiatric impairment and reduced quality of life.

Chapter 2: Phases and Foods of Sirtfood Diet

The Sirtfood Diet is focused on calorie restriction and the intake of a small number of foods. If you plan to follow the diet, you'll find that it's split up into two stages that last a total of 21 days—the first is seven days long, and the second is 14 days long. You can ingest just 1,000 calories a day over the first three days, which involves one meal as well as 3 Sirtfood green juices. The maximum calorie consumption is raised to 1,500 on days four and seven, and you're recommended to drink two green juices and eat two meals a day. The second phase of the diet includes 3 Sirtfood meals as well as a green juice every day. There is no calorie limit for the first 21 days, although you are advised to consume three meals rich in sirtfoods and a green juice each day if you wish to continue.

2.1 Foods to Eat On the Sirtfood Diet

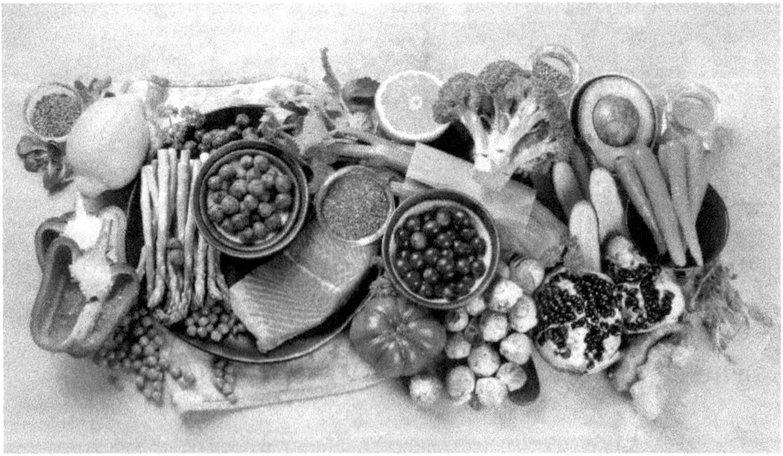

These are the top twenty foods that are said to raise the levels of sirtuins, which help your metabolism. For weight reduction, ten sections of sirtfoods are prescribed every day (the widest variety available, and therefore only two red wines - but nonetheless!) and 5 for maintenance.

1. **Bird's eye Chili,** they're often known as Thai chilies, and they're more strong and nutritious than standard chilies. Or use them to compliment sweet or sour foods.

2. **Buckwheat** is a type of grain. It's a fruit seed similar to rhubarb, but it's actually a pseudo-grain. Often available as soba (noodles), just make sure you have the wheat-free type.

3. **Capers** they're pickled flower buds, in case you are interested. They're perfect on salads or roasted cauliflower.

4. **Celery** If you're making a shake, don't throw out the hearts & leaves because they're the most nutritious.

5. **Cocoa** The flavonol-rich variety lowers blood pressure, blood sugar levels, and cholesterol. Look for a product with strong cocoa content.

6. **Coffee** Drink it black – there is some proof that milk can lessen sirtuin-activating nutrient absorption.

7. **Olive oil (extra virgin)** Extra virgin has more Sirt advantages as well as a more pleasing, peppery flavor.

8. Matcha or green tea Increase the absorption of sirtuin-producing nutrients by adding a slice of lemon. Matcha is much nicer; just make sure it's Japanese rather than Chinese to prevent lead poisoning.

9. Kale contains high levels of the sirtuin-activating nutrients quercetin as well as kaempferol. To serve as a salad, soak it with olive oil & lemon juice.

10. Lovage is a herb. It's a kind of herb. On a window ledge, cultivate your own and use it in stir-fries.

11. Medijool Dates They're a staggering 66 percent sugar, but when eaten in moderation, they don't increase blood sugar levels and have also been related to lower diabetes and heart disease rates.

12. Parsley is a herb. It's more than a garnish; it's even rich in apigenin. To get the best out of it, mix it into a smoothie or juice.

13. Chicory is a form of chicory that is the best color is red, but yellow can compensate. In a salad, toss it in.

14. Onion, red, the red type is healthier, and it's nice enough to consume raw. It can be chopped and added to a salad or eaten with a burger.

15. Red wine you've already heard of resveratrol, and the good thing is that it's heat-stable, meaning it can be used in cooking (as well as glugging it straight). The maximum concentration is found in Pinot noir.

16. Rocket Most of the least tainted salad greens on the market. Olive oil can be drizzled over it.

17. Soybeans and miso include a lot of sirtuin activators. Mix it into stir-fries.

18. Strawberries They're tasty but just have one teaspoon of sugar per 100 grams, according to a study, and they help the body tolerate sugary carbs.

19. Turmeric curcumin has anti-cancer properties, according to research. The body struggles to absorb it on its own, but boiling it in liquid and incorporating fat or black pepper improves absorption.

20. Walnuts Rich in fat and calories but well-known for lowering the risk of metabolic disorder. For a sirt-flavored pesto, mix them up with parsley.

Is the Stirfood diet efficient?

The developers of the Sirtfood Diet make ambitious promises, such as that it will boost weight loss, trigger your "skinny gene," and avoid diseases. The thing is that there isn't any evidence to back up these arguments. So far, there is no compelling proof that the Sirtfood Diet is more effective than every other calorie-restricted diet in terms of weight loss.

And, though most of these foods have health benefits, no long-term human studies have been conducted to assess if consuming a diet that is rich in sirtfoods has any significant health benefits. Nonetheless, the Sirtfood Diet focuses on the findings of a pilot study performed by the writers with 39 participants from their fitness center.

The participants adhered to the diet and exercised on a regular basis for one week. Participants shed a total of 7 pounds (3.2 kg) and retained or even developed muscle mass through the end of the week.

These findings, though, are hardly unexpected. Limiting your calorie consumption to 1,000 calories a day and walking at the same time would almost always result in weight loss.

Regardless, this form of fast weight loss is hardly genuine nor long-term, and this research did not track participants beyond the first week to see whether they gained some of the weight back, as is normal.

When you are drained of nutrients, the body uses up its emergency energy supplies, or glycogen, in addition to consuming fat and muscle. To be processed, each molecule of glycogen needs 3–4 molecules of water. When the body depletes glycogen, it also depletes this water. It's referred to as "water weight."

Just about one-third of the weight reduction during the first week of severe calorie restriction comes from fat, while the other two-thirds coming from water, muscle, and glycogen.

If you boost your calorie consumption, the body regenerates its glycogen reserves, and the weight returns.

Unfortunately, this form of calorie restriction will cause your body's metabolic growth to decrease, forcing you to eat far fewer calories a day for energy than before. This plan will most certainly help you shed a few pounds at first, but they will most likely return after the diet is done.

In terms of disease prevention, three weeks is possibly not sufficient enough to have any meaningful long-term effects. Including sirtfoods in your daily diet, on the other hand, might be a smart choice in the long run. But, in that situation, you may as well ignore the diet and get started right away.

2.2 Phases of Sirtfood Diet

The Sirtfood Diet is split into two phases, each lasting three weeks. After that, keep "sirtifying" the diet by adding as many sirtfoods as feasible into your meals.

The first phase- Green juices phase

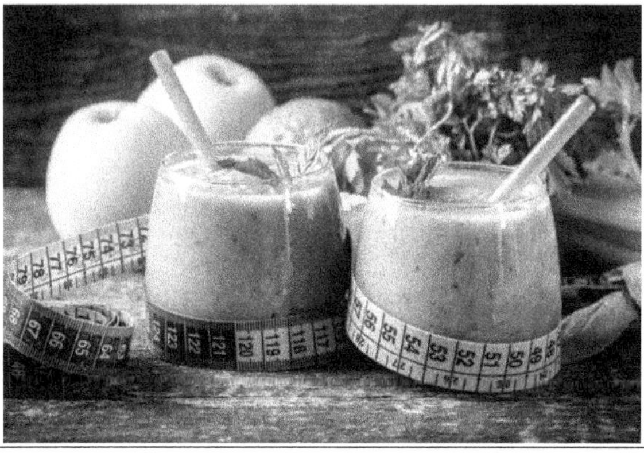

The first phase lasts seven days and entails calorie restriction as well as plenty of green juice. It focuses on helping you drop 7 pounds (3.2 kg) in seven days and is meant to jump-start the weight loss.

Caloric consumption is reduced to 1,000 calories over the first three days of phase one. You consume three green juices a day in addition to one meal. You may select from a variety of recipes in the book each day, all of which include sirtfoods as a main dish. The calorie consumption is raised to 1,500 calories on days 4–7 in phase one. This contains two green drinks a day and two main sirtfood-rich meals from the book.

Alcohol is strictly forbidden in Phase 1, and you must eliminate it at all costs. You can, though, drink as much tea, coffee, or green tea as you want. Just keep in mind that whether you incorporate sugar or milk into your tea or coffee, you'll be adding more calories to your diet. Be sure you don't go over your calorie limit.

The second phase- Maintenance phase

The second process lasts two weeks. You can begin to lose weight consistently through this "maintenance" phase.

For this step, there is no set calorie limit. Instead, you consume three sirtfood meals and one green juice every day. The dishes are yet again taken from the book's recipes. You can also consume 2-3 glasses of red wine a week, as well as, much water, coffee, tea, and green tea as you want.

After the diet

You should replicate these two steps as much as you like during the diet to lose more weight.

After following these steps, you're advised to keep "sirtifying" your diet by having sirtfoods in your meals on a regular basis. Sirtfoods may also be added to the diet as a snack or in existing foods.

You're even advised to start consuming the green juice on a regular basis. You'll have other berries, such as raspberries and blackberries, in your fruit intake in addition to strawberries. Instead of staying to walnuts, pistachios & peanuts are also delicious snacks. The Sirtfood Diet, therefore, becomes a dietary adjustment rather than a one-time diet.

Is sirtfood the new super-food?

There's no doubt that sirtfoods are beneficial to your health. They're typically rich in nutrients and filled with beneficial plant compounds. Furthermore, many of the items suggested on the Sirtfood Diet have been linked to health benefits in research.

Consuming moderate quantities of dark chocolate with a high cocoa content, for example, can help reduce the risk of heart disease and inflammation.

Green tea can reduce blood pressure and reduce the risk of stroke and diabetes.

Turmeric has several anti-inflammatory effects that favor the body as a whole and can also guard against chronic inflammation-related diseases. In reality, the plurality of sirtfoods is said to be beneficial to human health.

However, there is only tentative proof that rising sirtuin protein levels have health benefits. However, experiments on animals as well as cell lines have shown promising findings. Increased amounts of some sirtuin proteins, for example, have been linked to a longer lifetime in yeast, insects, and mice.

Sirtuin proteins often tell the body to burn extra fat for energy and increase insulin sensitivity while fasting or calorie restriction. Excessive sirtuin levels are linked to fat loss in mice in one study. Sirtuins will also play a role in lowering inflammation, inhibiting tumor growth, and delaying the progression of heart disease and Alzheimer's disease, according to some evidence.

While experiments in mice and human cell lines have yielded promising findings, no human studies on the consequences of growing sirtuin levels have been performed. As a result, it's unclear if growing sirtuin protein levels in the body would contribute to a longer lifetime or a reduced cancer risk in humans.

The production of compounds that raise sirtuin levels in the body is currently being investigated. In this way, human research on the impact of sirtuins on human health may begin. It would be unable to assess the consequences of elevated sirtuin levels before then.

Is it safe and long-term?

Sirtfoods are mostly healthy options, and their antioxidant and anti-inflammatory effects can also have certain health benefits. However, a small number of extremely nutritious foods would not serve to satisfy all of the body's dietary requirements.

The Sirtfood Diet is too restrictive and does not have any simple, distinct health benefits over other diets. Furthermore, consuming just 1,000 calories under the supervision of a practitioner is usually not advised. For certain individuals, also consuming 1,500 calories a day is too restrictive.

Having a drink of up to three green juices a day is also part of the diet. While juices can be a great source of minerals and vitamins, they are also high in sugar and lack the nutritious fiber found in whole fruits and vegetables.

Furthermore, drinking juice continuously during the day is harmful to both the blood sugar including your teeth. Not to mention that, since the diet is so restricted in terms of calories and food options, it is likely to be deficient in nutrition, vitamins, & minerals, particularly in the first phase. The regular recommended amount of protein, for example, ranges from 2 to 6 1/2 ounce equivalents and is determined by a number of variables, including:

- Regardless of whether you're a man or a woman
- How old are you?
- How productive are you?

This diet can be impossible to follow for the full three weeks due to the reduced calorie amounts and restricted food options.

When you weigh in the high initial costs of a juicer, the book, and some uncommon and costly ingredients, and also the time investment needed to cook particular meals and juices, this diet seems unfeasible and impractical for many individuals.

2.3 Pros and Cons of Sirtfood Diet

The Pros of Sirtfood Diet

- Many individuals would be enticed by the possibility of dropping a significant amount of weight in just three weeks.
- The eating plan promotes a number of polyphenol-rich ingredients that are often excellent sources of vitamins, minerals, and dietary fiber and will be suitable for the use of a variety of weight-loss diets or as part of a healthy, well-balanced diet.
- If a weight loss diet completes sustained total normal energy restriction, it would be effective. So the best advantage of the

Sirtfood diet is the normal energy limitation – if you adhere to it, you'll lose weight.

- Excluding high-energy, ultra-processed "junk" foods can also tend to reduce the risk of chronic disease.

However, there are certain disadvantages to remember.

The Cons of Sirtfood Diet

- Some of the foods included, like red wine and chocolate, should be consumed in smaller portions.
- Phase one, like most stringent diets, can be difficult, and it's not advised for individuals with chronic health problems unless they're under the care of a doctor.
- Instead of being all body fat, the accelerated weight reduction in the first step would be due to a loss of fluids and glycogen, the nutrition retained in muscles and the liver.
- Gallstones and amenorrhoea may also be caused by rapid weight loss (missing menstrual periods).
- Unique foods, like lovage, a European leafy green plant that leaves may be used as a herb, roots as a vegetable, and seeds as a seasoning, are included on the food list. Any of the other things on the list are pricey.

Everyone who is concerned about attempting the SirtFood diet should first consult with their physician. They will help them figure out if the diet is good for them by giving them recommendations and guidance.

The SirtFood diet is backed by supporters who say it assists in weight reduction, anti-aging, and disease prevention. However, since research on its efficacy is minimal, an individual should undertake this diet with precautions.

Chapter 3: Recipes of sirtfood diet

The Sirtfood diet entails eating a lot of "sirtfoods." These foods function by activating particular proteins in the body called sirtuins, according to the diet's creators. They are thought to help prevent cells in the body from dying while they are stressed, as well as control inflammation, metabolism, the aging process and the weight loss. Following are some delicious and tasteful recipes you can enjoy in your breakfast, lunch, dinner and snacks.

1. SIRTFOOD DIET GREEN JUICE

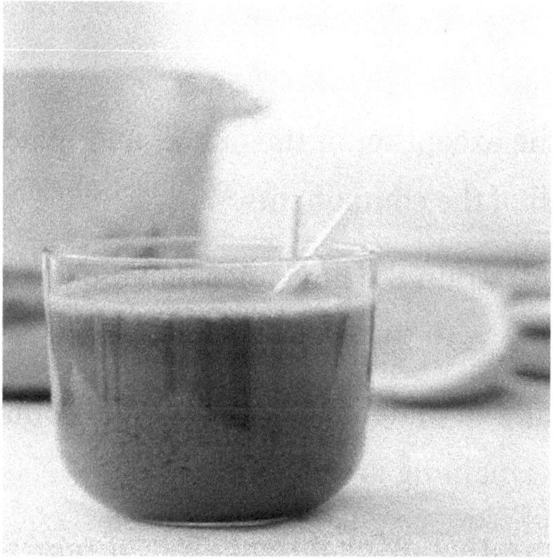

Serving: 1

Preparation time: 5 minutes

Nutritional values: Calories-101kcal|Carbs-21g|Protein-5g|Fat-1g

Ingredients

- Kale (75 g)
- 5 g parsley
- 30 g rocket
- A couple of celery sticks
- 1/2 apple (green)
- 1 cm of ginger
- 1/2 lemon juice
- 1/2 tsp. matcha green tea

Directions

1. With the exception of the lemon and matcha green tea, juice all of the components.
2. By hand, strain the lime juice into the green juice.
3. In a container, add a small quantity of green juice and whisk in the matcha. Transfer to the container and stir in the remaining green juice.
4. You can either drink it right away or reserve it for later.

2. GREEN JUICE IN THE BLENDER

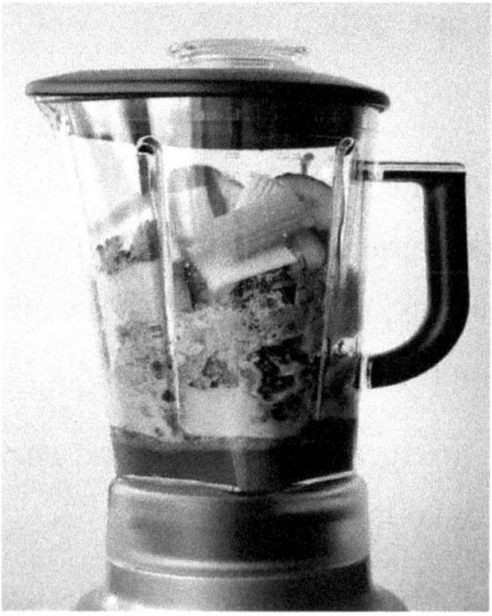

Serving: 4

Preparation time: 10 minutes

Nutritional values: Calories-105kcal|Carbs-22g|Protein-5g|Fat-2g

Ingredients

- 1 1/2 cup of water
- Kale, 2 cups
- 2 cored green apples
- Parsley leaves, 1/2 cup
- 1 quartered medium cucumber
- 2 stalks of celery, chopped roughly

- 1 chopped ginger piece (1 inch)
- Lemon extract, 2 tbsp.

Directions

1. Place all of the ingredients in the blender jug in the sequence specified above. Blend on the maximum level, such as "liquefy," before the juice is well-blended. (It will have a smoothie-like consistency.)
2. Place the mixture into bottles and serve if you like to consume the pulp with the juice.
3. Pour the mixture into a fine-mesh sieve and press the pulp through the sieve with a spatula to remove as much liquid as feasible if you want a finer consistency.
4. Fill glasses halfway with the strained juice and serve.

3. GREEN JUICE SALAD

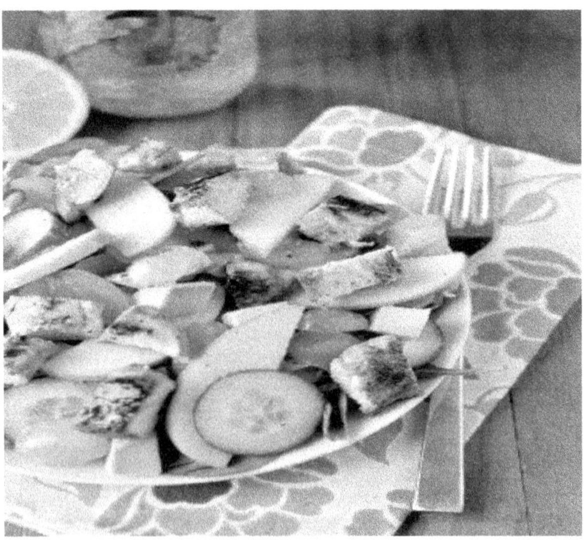

Serving: 1

Preparation time: 10 minutes

Nutritional values:

Ingredients

- 1/2 lemon juice
- 1 cm grated ginger
- Salt & pepper to taste.
- 1 tbsp. olive oil
- 2 kale handfuls, sliced
- 1 rocket, handful (arugula)
- 1 tbsp. fresh parsley
- 2 sliced celery sticks
- 1/2 sliced green apples
- 6 halves of walnut

Directions

1. Shake together the lemon juice, ginger, salt, pepper, and olive oil in a Jam-jar.
2. Pour the dressing over the kale in a wide mixing dish. For 1 minute, compress the dressing into the kale.
3. Mix with all of the remaining products properly.

4. SUPER GREEN TEA SMOOTHIE

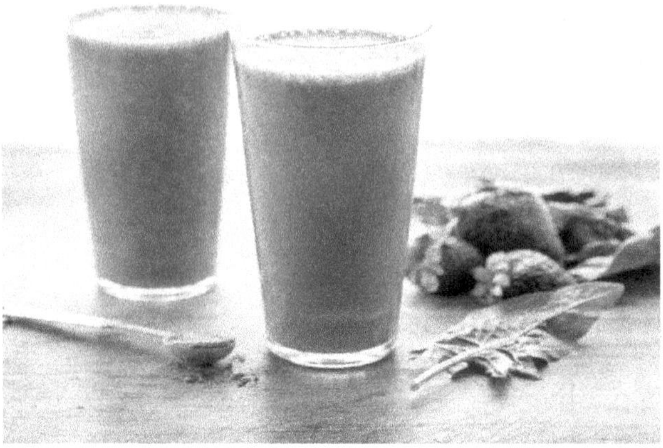

Serving: 3

Preparation time: 5 minutes

Nutritional values: Calories-200kcal|Carbs-29g|Protein-14g|Fat-1g

Ingredients

- 1 cup almond milk (unsweetened)
- 1/2 sliced banana
- 1 cup fresh spinach leaves, loosely packed
- 1 cup hulled strawberries
- 3/4 cup hulled strawberries
- 1 tbsp. vanilla protein powder (depending on the brand) 1 serving

- Half teaspoon of matcha powder

Directions

1. In a blender, mix together almond milk, banana, spinach, bananas, ice, protein powder, and matcha powder.
2. Puree at fast speed for 45 seconds, or until absolutely smooth, as well, as ice is no longer chunky.

5. SIRTFOOD FRIENDLY CHICKPEA CURRY

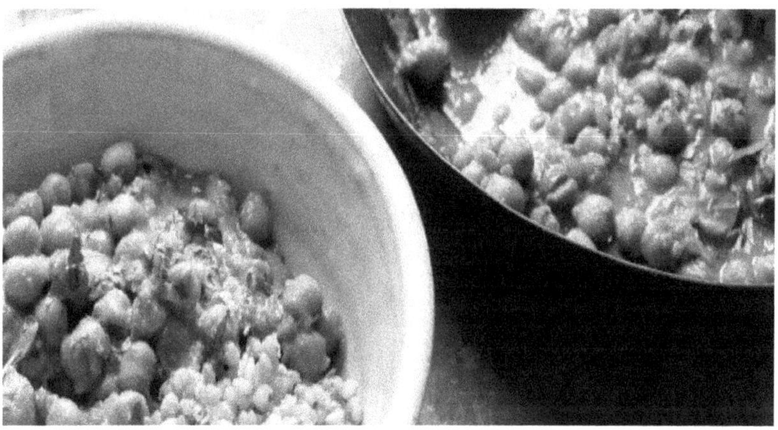

Serving: 4

Preparation time: 50 minutes

Nutritional values: Calories-500kcal|Carbs-15g|Protein-6g|Fat-10g

Ingredients

- 1 tablespoon of coconut oil
- 1 sliced onion, red

- 3 finely minced garlic cloves
- 1 inch of finely sliced fresh ginger
- 1-2 minced Birdseye chilies
- Curry powder, 1 tablespoon
- 1 tablespoon cumin powder
- 1 tablespoon turmeric powder
- 3 vine-ripened tomatoes
- 2 cups of vegetable broth
- Kale, 3 oz.
- 2 cans of chickpeas (15 oz.) processed and dried
- 2 tbsp. coriander, finely chopped
- 1/2 cup yogurt (plain)
- Buckwheat, 10 oz.

Directions

1. Fry it up. Over moderate flame, heat a large saucepan. Fry the onion, garlic, ginger, also chilies in coconut oil for 2–3 minutes. Integrate the curry and cumin powder, and 1/2 tbsp. Turmeric in a mixing bowl. Cook for another 1–2 minutes over low–medium flame.
2. Cut and prepare. Each tomato should be cut into 1/2-inch wedges. Make an attempt to hold quite enough juice as

feasible. Cook for 1–2 minutes after adding them to the saucepan.

3. Toss in the ingredients. Bring the stock, chickpeas, and kale to a boil, then reduce to a simmer for 7–8 minutes.
4. Buckwheat should be cooked. Cook the buckwheat as per the box directions while the curry is cooking. In the water you're preparing in, stir in the remaining turmeric.
5. Combine the coriander then yogurt in a mixing bowl. Transfer the coriander as well as yogurt to the curry until the kale is tender. Get it to a simmer, and switch off the stove. Serve with buckwheat.

6. LEMON GARLIC SAUTEED KALE

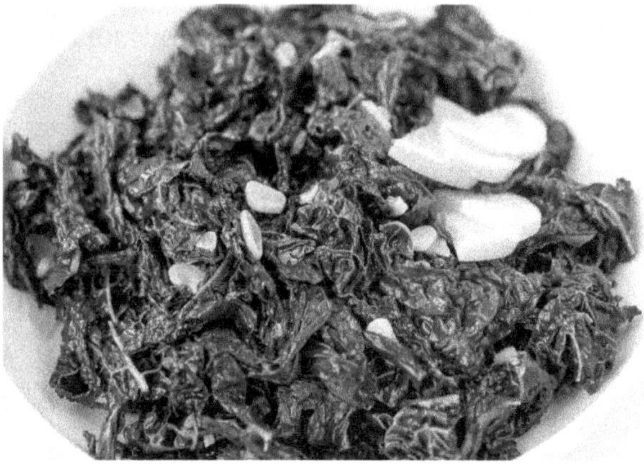

Serving: 4

Preparation time: 20 minutes

Nutritional values: Calories-118kcal|Carbs-4g|Protein-2g|Fat-2g

Ingredients

- 3 tbsp. extra-virgin olive oil
- 3 garlic cloves, peeled and diced
- Pinch of red pepper flakes
- 1 kale bunch, large (7 - 8 cups diced leaves)
- Half cup stock, white wine, or water, plus additional as required
- 1/4 tsp. fine sea salt, or more if desired
- Half lemon

Directions

1. Remove the leaves from the stems after rinsing the kale. Remove the stems and discard or preserve them to use in homemade stock later. Chop the kale leaves coarsely into 2-inch fragments that are arbitrarily shaped.
2. In a large skillet, melt the olive oil over moderate flame. Bring the garlic and red pepper flakes as the oil begin to shimmer. Cook, frequently mixing, until the garlic softens but does not brown.
3. Combine the sliced stock, kale leaves, and 1/4 tsp. in a wide mixing bowl. Cook, turning the kale across the pan periodically, for 7 to 8 minutes, or until bright green, tender, and wilted. If the liquid disappears until the kale is soft, bring a little more to the skillet.

4. Taste and season with more salt if necessary, then stir in half a lemon juice to finish.

7. SMOKED SALMON OMELET

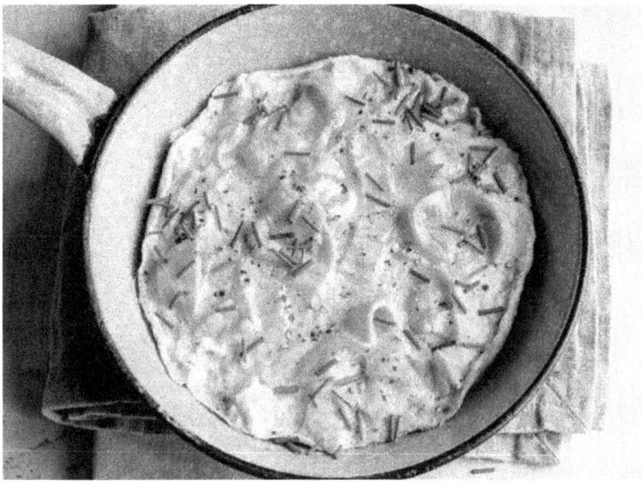

Serving: 1

Preparation time: 10 minutes

Nutritional values: Calories-274kcal|Carbs-5g|Protein-23g|Fat-17

Ingredients

- 2 eggs, large
- 1 tbsp. fresh herbs (at least 2 or 3 different herbs are preferred) (like parsley, tarragon, thyme, chives, etc.)
- 1/4 tsp. of kosher salt
- 1/4 tsp. of black pepper, freshly ground
- 2 slices of smoked salmon

- Lemon wedge
- A half tsp. of capers
- 1 tsp. creme fraiche or sour cream
- For garnish, Chives

Directions

1. Integrate the eggs, herbs, salt, and pepper in a tiny bowl. Mix until foamy and well blended.
2. For around 30 seconds, prepare a tiny skillet over medium-high heat. Spray the plate liberally with vegetable spray. In the pan, pop the eggs.
3. Lift the pan 1-2" above the blaze and swirl the pan to brush the bottom part with the mixture of the egg. Pull one side of the omelet apart from the pan with a spatula when simultaneously lowering the pan to another side, so the raw egg runs into and occupies the empty room. Repeat this process until the eggs are somewhat fried. Remove the pan from the heat.
4. Cover the omelet in half or thirds with the spatula (sort of folding it over on itself). Cover with smoked salmon, capers, creme fraiche, and chives after slipping the omelet onto a tray. Serve with a lemon wedge.

8. ARUGULA PESTO

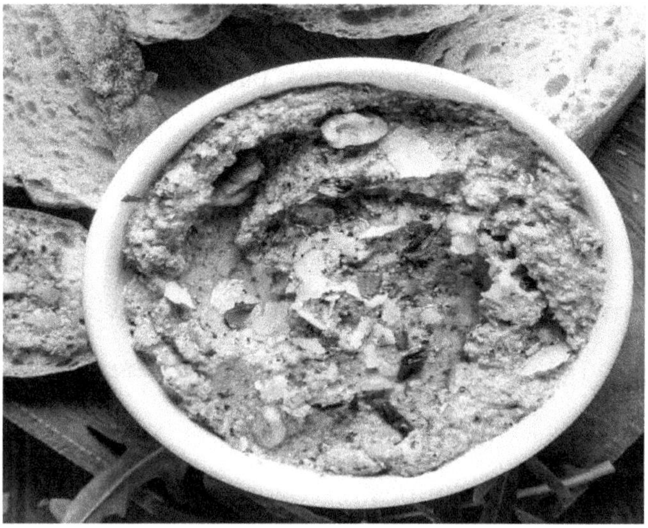

Serving: 2

Preparation time: 6 minutes

Nutritional values: Calories-158kcal|Carbs-2g|Protein-3g|Fat-16g

Ingredients

- 4 cups of fresh arugula, packed
- Walnuts, 1/2 cup
- 1/2 cup grated cheese (Parmesan)
- 2 garlic cloves, chopped
- 2 tbsp. lemon juice
- To taste kosher salt
- 1/2 cup of extra virgin olive oil

Directions

1. In the bowl of a food processor, combine the arugula, walnuts, garlic, lemon juice, parmesan cheese, as well as salt (you can also use a blender). Pulse the mixture 5-10 times until it is evenly sliced and has developed a thick paste.
2. Scrounge down each side of the bowl with a spatula or spoon after turning off the food processor.
3. Slowly drizzle in the olive oil when the food processor is moving until the pesto reaches the perfect consistency. You won't use all of the oil – you can only use about a quarter of a cup – so pour it gradually and hold an eye on the pesto as it blends. Scrounge down each side of the food processor if necessary to ensure that all of the ingredients are evenly mixed into the pesto.
4. Serve right away or keep in the refrigerator for up to a week in an airtight container.

9. FRENCH FRIES WITH RANCH DIP (PALEO&WHOLE30)

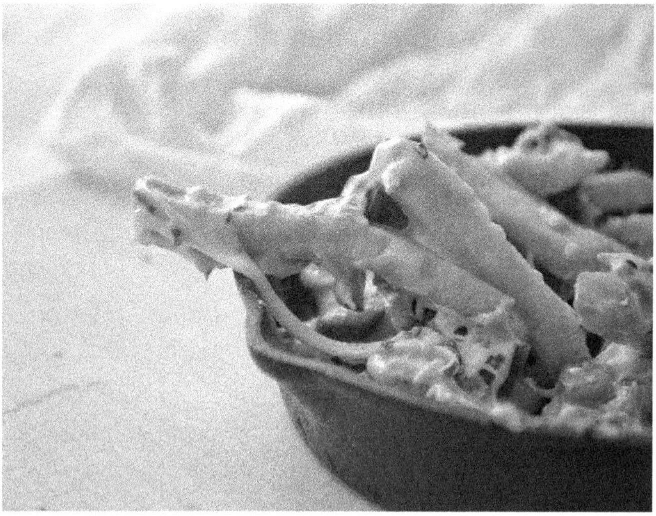

Serving: 6

Preparation time: 45 minutes

Nutritional values: Calories-342kcal|Carbs-15g|Protein-2g|Fat-30g

Ingredients

For Fries

- 2 peeled & rinsed russet potatoes
- 1 tablespoon avocado oil or olive oil with a mild flavor
- To taste, sea salt & pepper
- Optional: 1/4 teaspoon onion powder

For Ranch Dip

- 1 cup Paleo mayonnaise (homemade* or store-bought**)
- 1 tsp. chili powder, chipotle
- 1 teaspoon lime or lemon juice
- 1 1/2 teaspoon powdered onion
- 1 teaspoon powdered garlic
- 1 tsp. paprika (smoked)
- 2 tsp. chives (dried)
- salt for taste if desired

Directions

1. Preheat oven to 425°F. Line two wide baking sheets with parchment paper.
2. To remove as much moisture as practicable, cut the potatoes into half-inch "fries" and pat them dry on both sides with paper towels.
3. Toss the fries in a wide mixing bowl with the oil, salt, and pepper, as well as some onion powder if used. Ensure that the fries are well-coated with oil.
4. Spread the fries out uniformly on the two parchment-lined baking sheets, allowing a minimum 1/2 inch gap between them. More space means crispier fries!

5. Bake for 20 minutes at 425 degrees, then flip them (or shake them a little to make as much as possible), decrease the heat to 400 degrees, and bake for another 20 minutes, or until light brown and crispy.
6. Make the ranch whilst the fries are baking! In a medium pan, whisk together all of the ingredients and set aside until the fries are ready. If needed, serve with hot fries & fresh chopped chives. The chipotle ranch is also delicious with burgers, chili, chicken, and everything else! Have fun.

10. CHOCOLATE COVERED STRAWBERRY POPSICLES

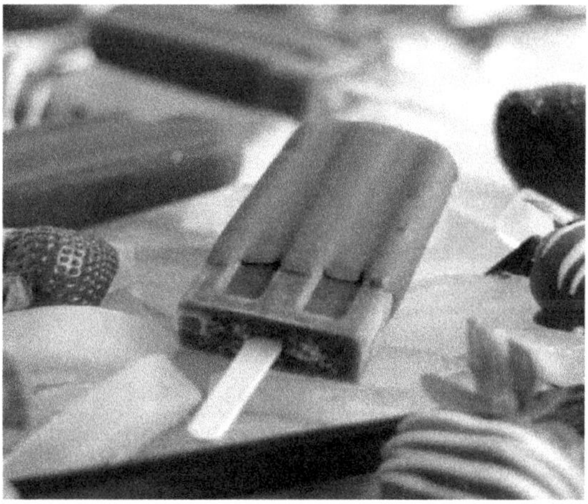

Serving: 7

Preparation time: 30 minutes

Nutritional values: Calories-250kcal|Carbs-32g|Protein-2g|Fat-13g

Ingredients

- 2 cups of fresh strawberries, quartered
- 4-5 bruised and quartered Medjool dates
- 1/4 cup of water
- Coconut cream (1/2 cup)
- 1/4 teaspoon of vanilla extract
- 1/4 teaspoon lemon extract, freshly squished
- 1/2 cup fresh strawberries, finely chopped (optional)

For Chocolate Coating:

- 1 cup sliced chocolate chips from a bar
- 2 tsp. coconut oil

Directions

1. Preheat a saucepan to medium-high heat.
2. Bring the dates, sugar, and 2 cups of quartered strawberries.
3. Simmer on low-medium heat for 10-15 minutes, or until the strawberries and dates crumble and the juices escape.
4. Switch off the flame, remove the medium-high heat, and put it aside to cool the strawberry-date-water mixture.
5. After the strawberry-date-water mixture has cooled, puree it with coconut cream, vanilla extract, & freshly squeezed lemon juice in a blender.

6. Cover a mixing bowl halfway with the ingredients of the blender. If using, add 1/2 cup finely sliced strawberries.
7. Place the Popsicle mixture in Popsicle molds and put it in the fridge overnight!
8. The strawberry cream popsicles would be wonderful as is at this stage. You might practically end here, but to take them to the next stage, let's Plunge them in dark chocolate!

For Chocolate Coating:

1. Place a baking sheet lined with parchment paper in the freezer before ready to use. This will keep the chocolate-covered popsicles cool as you focus on them.
2. Using the double broiler process, thoroughly melt the dark chocolate & coconut oil together. The melted chocolate must be ready to be poured. Take the pan off the heat and put it aside.
3. Work quickly for three popsicles at a time to prevent them from melting.
4. Three popsicles can be separated from the fridge mold. Set aside the covered baking sheet from the fridge. Dip the top half of each Popsicle into the molten chocolate. Please ensure the chocolate is well prepared before putting it on the cooled lined baking sheet. When you've finished all three popsicles, return the baking sheet to the freezer before

you're ready to make the next three. Working fast, repeat this process to cover the remaining popsicles.

5. If you've finished wrapping all of the popsicles in chocolate, place the baking sheet in the refrigerator to harden the chocolate shells before serving.
6. All leftover popsicles can be stored in an airtight freezer box with parchment paper between the layers of popsicles. Keep in the freezer and serve as needed!

11. SWEET POTATO SALAD WITH BACON

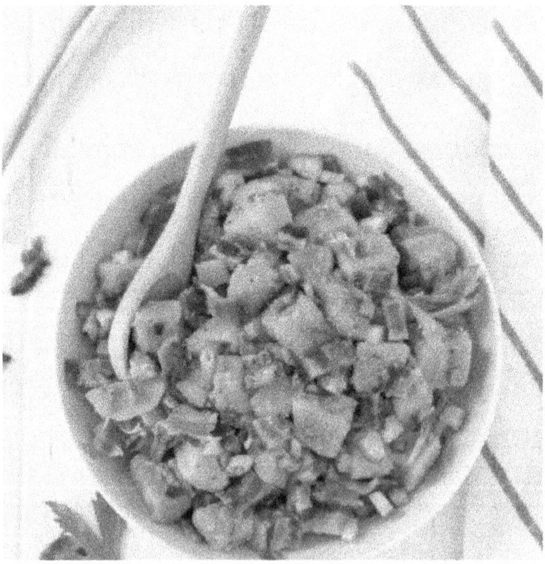

Serving: 6

Preparation time: 45 minutes

Nutritional values: Calories-222kcal|Carbs-23g|Protein-5g|Fat-13g

Ingredients

For Sweet Potato Salad:

- 4 thickly-cut bacon slices, cooked
- 3 large peeled sweet potatoes, cut into cubes
- 1 cup celery hearts, sliced thinly
- 1 cup green onions, sliced thinly

For Mustard Dressing:

- 2 tbsp. whole-grain mustard
- 1 jalapeno pepper, seeded as well as minced
- 2 minced garlic cloves
- 3 tbsp. rice vinegar
- 3 spoonful's of extra virgin olive oil
- 1/8 tsp. black pepper
- 1/4 tsp. kosher salt

Directions

1. Bring a large pot of salted water to a simmer before dropping in the sweet potatoes. Boil for 10 to 15 minutes, depending on the size of the potato chunks, until spoon tender. Drain, then soak with ice water softly and swiftly before setting aside.

2. Prepare the bacon using these simple instructions if necessary. Crush it into a significant mixing bowl once it has cooled. Combine the celery as well as green onions in a large mixing bowl.
3. Make the mustard dressing as follows: Mix the jalapeno (or Fresno chile), garlic, vinegar, mustard, olive oil, salt, as well as pepper together in a medium bowl or wide measuring cup.
4. Toss the sweet potatoes with the bacon in a bowl with the dressing, then softly toss to combine. Taste as well as season with salt and pepper as needed. Warm, chilled, or room temperature are all appropriate serving options.

12. PASTA SALAD

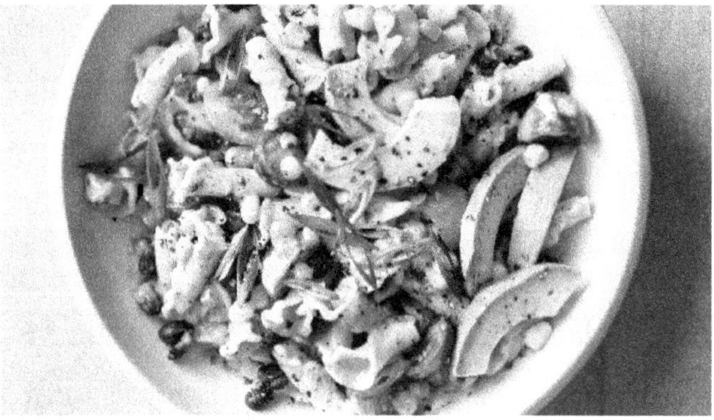

Serving: 6

Preparation time: 35 minutes

Nutritional values: Calories-400kcal|Carbs-39g|Protein-8g|Fat-25g

Ingredients

- 1 pound spiral pasta in three colors
- Salad seasoning mix, 6 tbsp.
- 1 bottle of Italian salad dressing (16 oz.)
- 1 (2.25 oz.) can of black olives, chopped
- 2 cups of cherry tomatoes
- 1 green bell pepper, thinly sliced
- Red bell pepper, finely chopped
- 1/2 yellow bell pepper, finely chopped

Directions

1. Cook pasta until al dente in a medium skillet of salted boiling water, then drain and wash under cold water.
2. Combine the salad spice mix as well as Italian dressing in a mixing bowl.
3. Toss the pasta with the cherry tomatoes, bell peppers, and olives in a salad bowl. Toss the salad with the dressing and chill overnight.

13. COFFEE ICECREAM

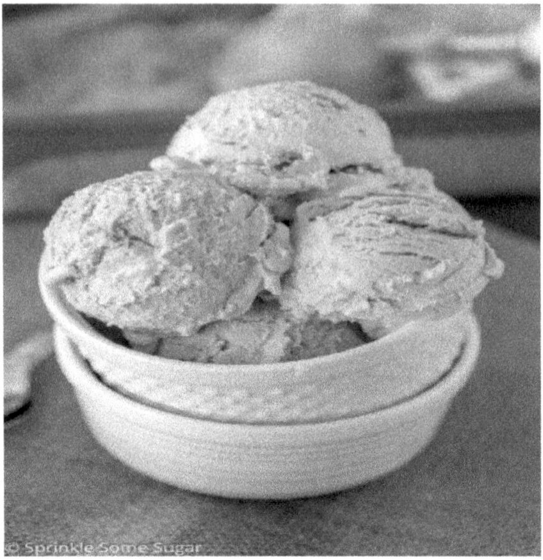

Serving: 5

Preparation time: 35 minutes

Nutritional values: Calories-182kcal|Carbs-9g|Protein-8g|Fat-13g

Ingredients

- 2 1/2 cup whole milk (600 ml)
- 1 1/2 cup granulated sugar (300 g)
- 1/8 teaspoon of salt
- 2 tbsp. decaffeinated instant coffee granules*
- 6 beaten egg yolks
- 2 1/4 cup heavy cream (540 ml)

- 1/2 tsp. extract of vanilla

Directions

1. Integrate the milk, sugar, salt, as well as coffee granules in a wide saucepan. Cook, stirring periodically, over a moderate flame until simmering. Turn down the heat to a low level.
2. In a small mixing bowl, gently pound the egg yolks. Pour half of the heated milk into the eggs slowly while whisking constantly. Transfer the blend to the container and cook, stirring periodically, over moderate flame unless thickened, around 5 minutes.
3. Using a fine-mesh sieve placed over a medium pot, drain the custard. To avoid a skin from emerging, cover it with plastic wrap that reaches the surface of the custard. Put it in the fridge until well chilled.
4. Whisk the cream as well as vanilla into the custard once smooth when prepared to make the ice cream. Following the manufacturer's directions, process the ice cream in an ice cream maker.
5. Serve promptly or put in a freezer-safe jar. The ice cream can be stored in the fridge for up to two weeks.

14. CASHEW CHICKEN SATAY SKEWERS WITH CHILI DIPPING SAUCE

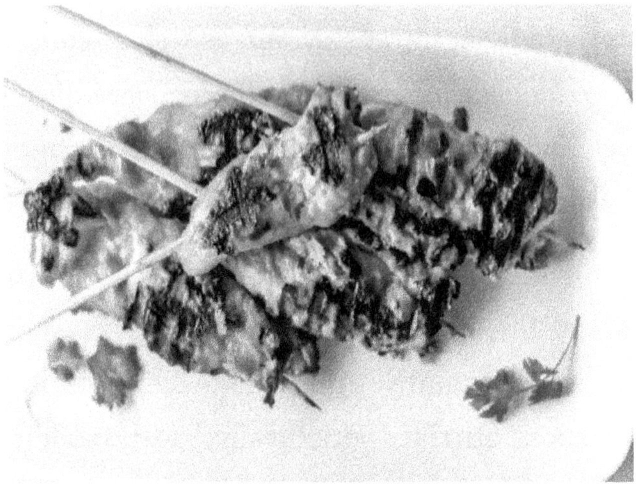

Serving: 4

Preparation time: 1hr 22min

Nutritional values: Calories-353kcal|Carbs-14g|Protein-25g|Fat-21g

Ingredients

- Half-cup of cashew butter
- Red chili paste, 2 tbsp.
- a 1/4 cup of pineapple juice
- 1 tablespoon coconut milk (full fat)
- 1 tsp. sesame oil
- coconut aminos, 1 tsp. (or soy sauce if not Whole30)

- 1 freshly squeezed lime
- A quarter teaspoon of salt
- 1 pound tenderloins of chicken
- 8 wooden skewers, drained
- Lime and cilantro for serving

Directions

1. In a mixing bowl, whisk together the cashew butter, pineapple juice, coconut milk, sesame oil, coconut aminos, red chili paste, lime juice, and salt. Mix thoroughly.
2. Place the chicken tenderloins in a large bowl or bag with half of the sauce. Allow marinating in the refrigerator for at least one hour and up to four hours.
3. Drench the skewers in water to prevent them from burning.
4. Enable the chicken to get to room temp on the counter thirty min before grilling.
5. Heat up the grill to moderate flame and skewer the chicken.
6. Before extracting the chicken, grill it for around 5-6 minutes per side.
7. Serve with extra lime and cilantro.

15. CINNAMON APPLE WRAPS

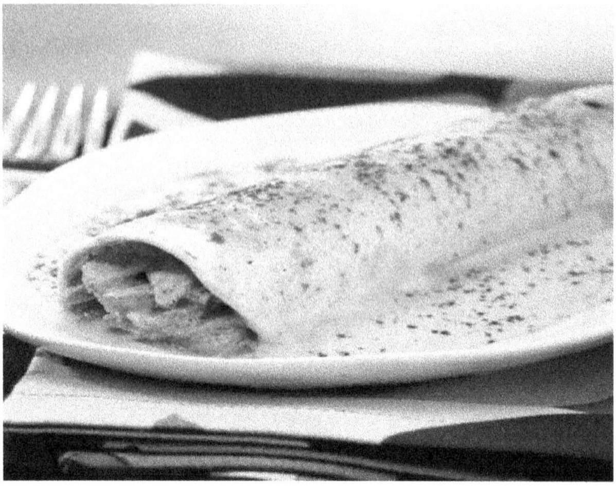

Serving: 2

Preparation time: 50 minutes

Nutritional values: Calories-603kcal|Carbs-65g|Protein-5g|Fat-36g

Ingredients

- 3/4 cup flour (all-purpose)
- 1/4 cup of shortening
- 1/2 tsp. salt
- 2 to 3 tbsp. ice-cold water
- 2 tbsp. Melted butter (divided)
- 2 tbsp. of sugar
- 1/2 tsp. cinnamon powder

- 1 large stripped and quartered apple

Directions

1. Incorporate flour and salt in a mixing bowl; slice in shortening unless crumbly. Toss with a fork as you gradually incorporate the water before a ball emerges. Roll out dough into a 10-inch square on a lightly floured surface and sprinkle with 1 tbsp. Butter. Fold the paper into thirds. Cut lengthwise into four stripes until rolling into a 10-in. x 6-in. rectangle. Using butter, cover the pan.
2. Half of the sugar & cinnamon mixture can be sprinkled over the strips. Put an apple wedge on each pastry layer and wrap it around the apple. Cover a baking sheet with cooking spray before covering it with foil.
3. Place the wraps on the pan that has been prepared. Brush with the remaining butter and top with the leftover cinnamon-sugar mixture. Preheat oven to 400°F and bake for 28-32 minutes, or until lightly browned. Serve hot.

16. HAWAIIAN SALAD

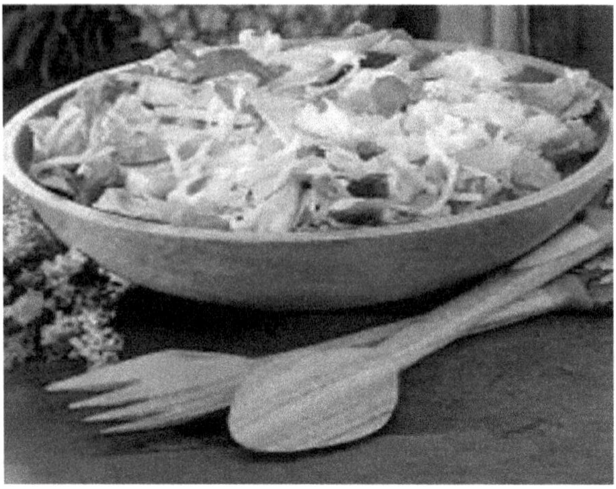

Serving: 6

Preparation time: 10 minutes

Nutritional values: Calories-237kcal|Carbs-9g|Protein-5g|Fat-20g

Ingredients

- 3/4 cup juiced pineapple tidbits
- 6–8 cups salad greens, torn
- 1 cup cheddar cheese, shredded
- Half cup of mayonnaise
- 1 tbsp. sugar

Directions

1. Drain the pineapple, retaining 1 tablespoon of the juice. Integrate the greens, pineapple, and cheese in a wide

mixing bowl. Whisk together the mayonnaise, sugar, and reserved pineapple juice in a small bowl. Toss the salad in the seasoning to coat.

17. SPICED BEEF BURGER

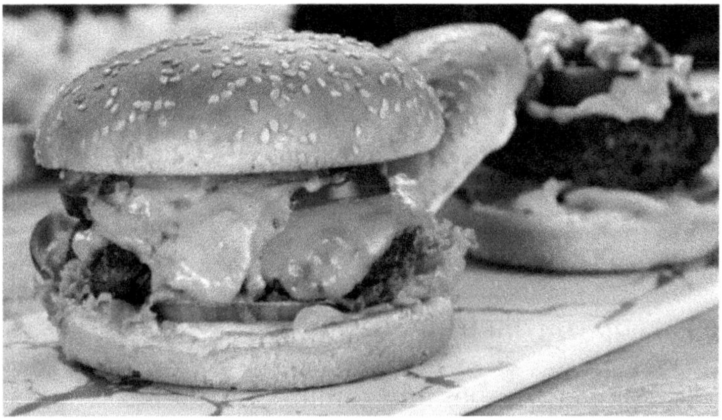

Serving: 4-6

Preparation time: 40 minutes

Nutritional values: Calories-317kcal|Carbs-20g|Protein-24g|Fat-15g

Ingredients

- 2 cloves of garlic
- 1 1/2 tsp. salt (kosher)
- 1 tsp. freshly grated ginger
- 1/4 cup onion, grated
- 1/4 tsp. cayenne pepper
- 2 tsp. coriander powder

- 2 tsp. cumin powder
- 1/2 tsp. allspice powder
- 1/2 tsp. black pepper
- 1/4 cup flat-leaf parsley, finely chopped
- 1/2 pound minced beef (at least 20% fat for a juicier burger)
- olive oil
- 3 pita bread slices
- 3/4 cup tzatziki from the store
- Slices of cucumber and tomato, butter lettuce, and mint leaves

Directions

1. Preheat a gas or barbecue grill to medium-high (400°) or a stovetop grill pan to moderate (400°).
2. Garlic should be minced with salt and pounded into a paste with the flat side of a knife. Scrape into a large mixing bowl and blend with ginger, onion, coriander, cumin, cayenne, allspice, pepper, and parsley.
3. Toss in the ground beef. Mix softly with your hands.
4. Form the mixture into 6 elongated patties, each about 3/4 inch thick, that will fit in a pita half. Use tongs and a pile of oiled paper towels, oil the cooking grate. Grill

patties for 4 to 5 minutes a side, or until well golden brown and only pink inside.

5. Halve the pita bread crosswise. To make pockets, remove the halves gently. Dust each with oil before putting it on the grill. The pita should be toasted for 1 to 2 minutes or until lightly golden and crisp. 1–2 tbsp. Tzatziki should be spread within each pocket. Within, tuck the burger, cucumber, cabbage, lettuce, then mint leaves.

18. CHICKEN PESTO ROLLS

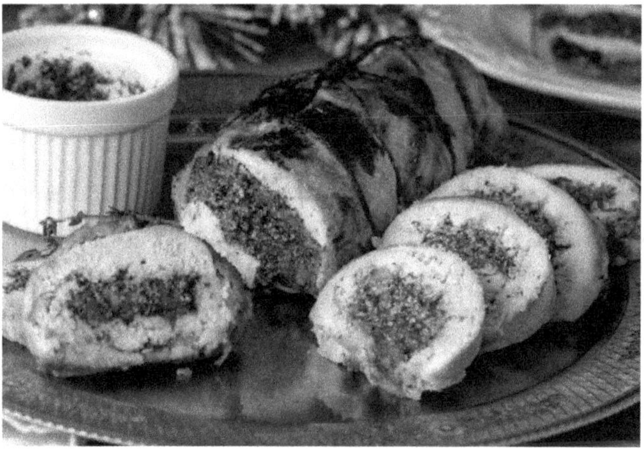

Serving: 8

Preparation time: 40 minutes

Nutritional values: Calories-295kcal|Carbs-3g|Protein-32g|Fat-16g

Ingredients

- 2-pound chicken breasts (four medium/large breasts)

- 1 tsp. (garlic) (or to taste)
- Black pepper, 1/4 teaspoon (or as per taste)
- Pesto sauce (1/2 cup) (about 8 Tbsp. total)
- 8 oz. sliced mozzarella cheese (reserve 2 oz. for topping)
- 2 medium tomatoes, thinly cut into 16 circles
- Optional: 1 cup of cherry tomatoes
- 1 tablespoon shredded fresh basil leaves as a garnish
- 1 tablespoon extra-virgin olive oil
- 1 tbsp. butter (unsalted)

Directions

1. Preheat the oven to 425 degrees Fahrenheit. Make 8 thin chicken cutlets by halving a chicken breast lengthwise. Pound each cutlet into 1/8" wide cutlets in a quart-size Ziploc bag and between two sheets of plastic wrap. Sprinkle garlic salt and black pepper on all sides of the chicken.
2. Spread 1 tablespoon pesto in the middle of each cutlet, then layer with 2 thin sliced tomatoes and 2-3 tablespoons mozzarella cheese. Roll the chicken tightly and use a toothpick to secure the ends.
3. Preheat a deep oven-safe pan over medium heat with 1 tablespoon oil and 1 tablespoon butter. Braise the

chicken roll-ups on both sides unless golden (4 min each side or 8 min total on the stove).

4. Cover with the leftover cheese as well as 1 cup of cherry tomatoes. Bake at 425°F for 13-15 minutes (13 minutes for moderate chicken breasts and 15 minutes for larger chicken breasts), or until the internal temperature of the chicken exceeds 160°F on an instant-read thermometer.

19. BUCKWHEAT PIZZA WITH ROCKET PESTO ROASTED MUSHROOM AND GARLIC BUTTER

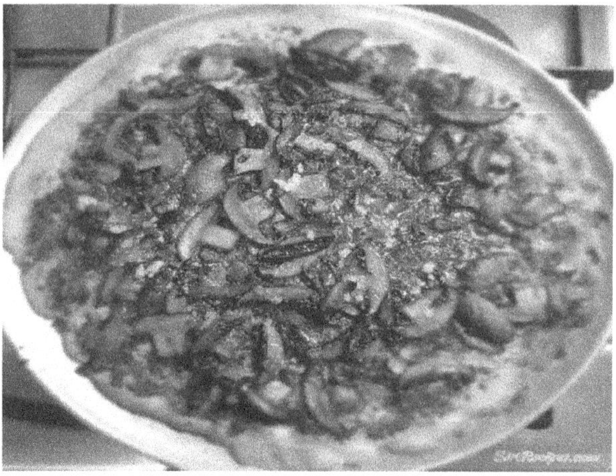

Serving: 4

Preparation time: 1 hour

Nutritional values: Calories-260kcal|Carbs-27g|Protein-7g|Fat-14g

Ingredients

For Buckwheat Pizza:

- 7 g yeasts, dry
- 1 teaspoon brown sugar
- 200 grams buckwheat flour
- 300 mL warm water
- 200 g whole-wheat flour
- 1 tablespoon of extra virgin olive oil

For Rocket Pesto:

- 1 cup leaves of rocket
- 1 cup parsley, flat-leaf
- 1 cup fresh basil
- Extra virgin olive oil, 1/3 cup
- 1 teaspoon coriander powder
- 1 teaspoon mustard seeds
- Walnuts (20 g)
- 2 cloves garlic, minced pinch salt, and pepper to taste

For Mushrooms, Roasted

- Shiitake mushrooms (200 g)
- Extra virgin olive oil, 1.5 tbsp.
- 2 minced garlic cloves
- 1 finely sliced brown onion

- pinch of salt & pepper to taste
- Butter and garlic
- 4 tablespoons ghee (or unsalted butter)
- 2 minced garlic cloves

Directions

For Buckwheat Pizza:

1. In a small bowl, mix the yeast & sugar in the water. Protect with a tea towel, then set aside for 10 to 15 minutes.
2. Trawl the flours together in a mixing bowl. Mix the yeast mixture & oil into the flour to form a dough.
3. Knead unless soft and flexible, then move to an oiled bowl, protect with a hygienic damp tea towel, and set aside for 45-60 min, or until increased in size. Meanwhile, make the pesto and the mushrooms (see instruction below).
4. Preheat the oven to 230°C/gas 8 and set aside. Knead the dough once more to extract the air. Divide the dough in half and roll out 1 piece of dough into a circle on a lightly floured surface. Put on a pizza stone or a nonstick baking tray that has been oiled.

5. Cover the dough with a thin coat of pesto, leaving a space around the edge for the crust, then cover with roasted mushrooms.
6. Leave for 15-20 minutes prior to baking to allow the dough to rise again, resulting in a lighter base.
7. Bake about 10-12 minutes.
8. Put on a cutting board after removing it from the oven. Brush the garlic butter over the crust and serve.

For Rocket Pesto:

1. Prepare an ice bath and get a pan of salted water to a boil. Boil the basil, parsley, and arugula for 30 seconds, then move to an ice bath for 1 minute to cool. Wiggle the greens to extract any extra liquid before mixing them with the residual pesto ingredients in a blender.
2. Set aside after puréeing until smooth.

For Mushrooms, Roasted:

1. Set the oven to 200 degrees Celsius. Integrate the mushrooms, olive oil, garlic, onion, salt, & pepper on a baking sheet and toss to coat.
2. Cook, mixing halfway through, for 20 minutes, or until soft and golden brown. Place aside.

For Butter and Garlic:

1. Take the butter & garlic to a boil in a medium saucepan. Cook unless aromatic, around 1 to 2 minutes; just don't let it burn. Set aside after removing from the heat.

20. CHICKEN AND BROCCOLI STIR FRY

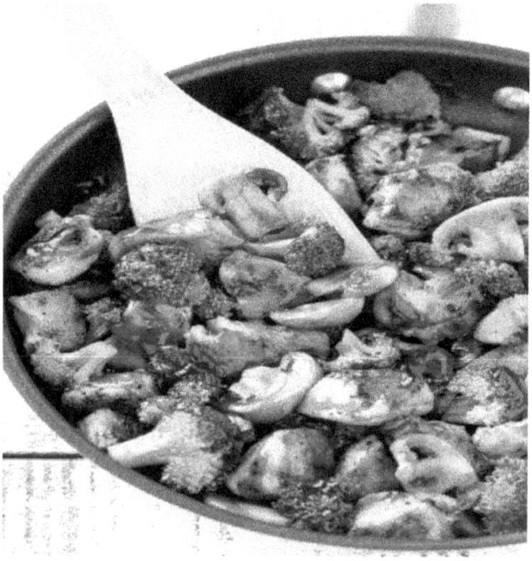

Serving: 4

Preparation time: 35 minutes

Nutritional values: Calories-351kcal|Carbs-26g|Protein-34g|Fat-13g

Ingredients

- 1 tbsp. egg white (approximately 1/2 medium egg white)
- 1 tbsp. mirin (rice wine) or sherry (dry)
- Cornstarch, 3 tbsp.

- 1 pound chicken breasts, skinless and boneless, sliced into 1/2-inch chunks
- 1/4 cup of oyster sauce
- 2 broccoli bunches, thick stems stripped and sliced into bits
- 2 tbsp. extra-virgin olive oil
- 3 garlic cloves, finely chopped
- 1 tablespoon peeled ginger, finely chopped
- 1 bunch finely chopped scallions
- Four to five baby bell peppers, cut into thin rings (any color)
- 1 or 2 seeded and finely chopped red jalapeno peppers
- 1/4 cup toasted diced almonds or diced cashews

Directions

1. Boil some water in a large pot. In a medium bowl, mix together the egg white, mirin, and 1 tbsp. Cornstarch. Toss in the chicken to coat it. In a medium bowl, combine the remainder 2 tbsp. Cornstarch, the oyster sauce, and 1/2 cup water.
2. Cook the broccolini in the boiling water for 1 to 2 minutes, or until crisp-tender. Drain and wash well with cool water.

3. In a wide nonstick skillet, melt 1 tbsp. Oil over medium heat. Cook, stirring periodically, until the chicken is no longer pink, around 4 minutes. Place on a plate to cool. Turn the heat up to maximum and pour in the remaining 1 tbsp. of olive oil. Stir in the ginger and garlic for 30 seconds. Mix in the scallions and peppers for another minute. Stir in the chicken, broccolini, and nuts for another 2 minutes.
4. Turn down the heat to moderate and add the oyster sauce blend to the skillet, whisking continuously. Cook, constantly stirring, for 3 minutes, or until the sauce has thickened.

21. ZEBRA BREAD WITH CREAM CHEESE

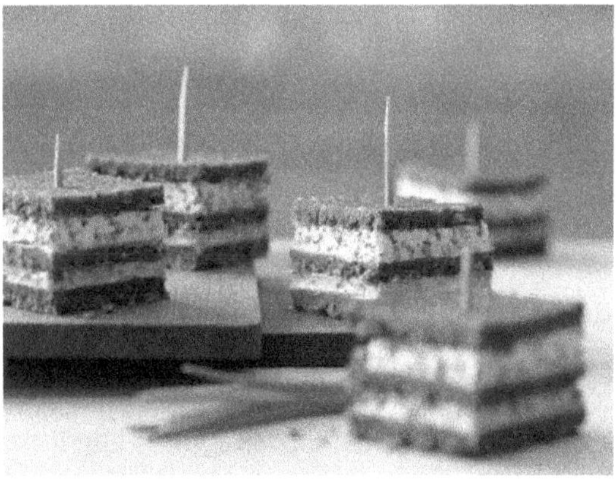

Serving: 12

Preparation time: 15 minutes

Nutritional values: Calories-60kcal|Carbs-8g|Protein-3g|Fat-2g

Ingredients

- 1/2 bunch of chives
- Cream cheese, 6 ounces (13 percent fat)
- Salt & peppers
- 1 tsp. paprika powder
- Pumpernickel bread, 6 slices

Directions

1. Rinse and pat dry the chives. Make tiny rings out of it.
2. Add a pinch of salt & pepper to the cream cheese. Cream cheese should be divided into 2 bowls.
3. Mix the chives into one of the cream cheese bowls. Combine the leftover cream cheese with the paprika.
4. Put the chive-cream cheese combination thickly on two pumpernickel slices. Layer the paprika-cream cheese thickly on the remaining 2 pumpernickel slices.
5. Place a paprika strip on top of a chive slice, then add a plain pumpernickel slice on top. Repeat with the remaining bread slices. Press down the stacks
6. 6 toothpicks, evenly spaced, can be used to hold the stacks. Each stack can be cut into 6 blocks.

22. SPAGHETTI WITH TOMATOES AND ZUCCHINI

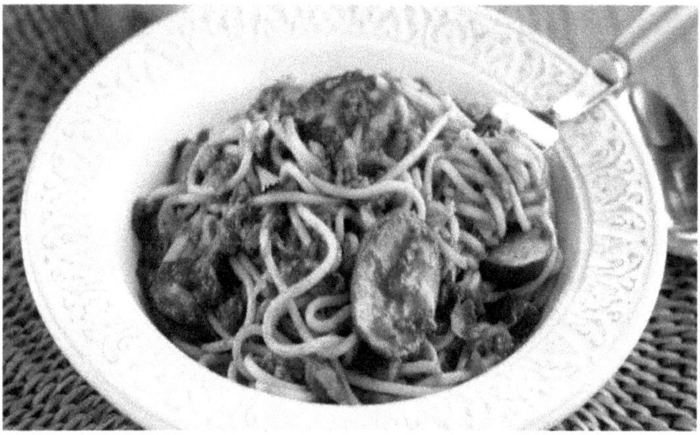

Serving: 4-6

Preparation time: 50 minutes

Nutritional values: Calories-369kcal|Carbs-51g|Protein-15g|Fat-14g

Ingredients

- Kosher salt.
- 1 zucchini (medium) cut into thin circles
- 1 standard size yellow summer squash, thinly sliced
- Cherry tomatoes, 1 pint
- 1 fennel bulb, cut, cored, and sliced thinly
- 1/2 finely minced onion
- 4 garlic cloves, minced
- 2 tbsp. fresh oregano, minced

- Half-cup of extra-virgin olive oil
- 1/2 teaspoon crushed red pepper flakes
- Pepper, freshly ground
- 1 lb. spaghetti
- 1 lemon's juice
- Topping: grated parmesan cheese

Directions

1. Set the oven to 450 degrees Fahrenheit. Boil a large container of salted water.
2. In a wide mixing bowl, mix the zucchini, yellow squash, fennel, onion, tomatoes, garlic, and oregano. Toss in the olive oil, red pepper flakes, and a pinch of salt and pepper to taste.
3. Transfer the mixture uniformly between two baking sheets. Roast for 15 to 25 minutes, or until the squash as well as other vegetables tend to caramelize. Scrounge the veggies into a wide mixing bowl and place a plate on top to stay warm.
4. By now, the pasta water should really be heating. Stir in the spaghetti to split the strands. Cook until the pasta is al dente, around 8 or 9 minutes, then rinse.
5. Integrate the spaghetti and the vegetable mix in a large mixing bowl. Toss all together with a squeeze of lemon

juice. Distribute among the bowls. If needed, garnish with Parmesan.

23. PUMPKIN PASTA WITH ARUGULA AND CHICKEN

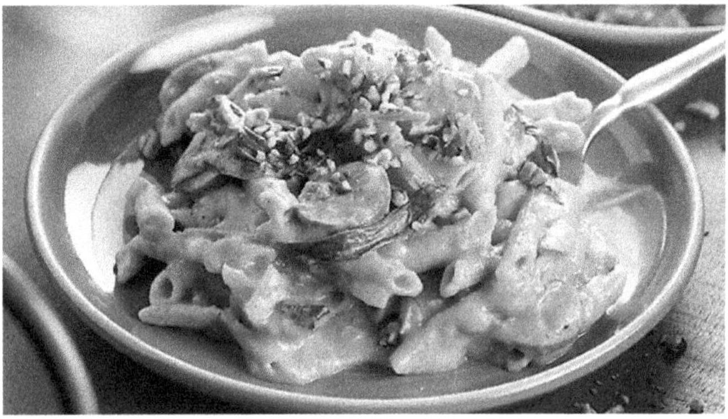

Serving: 4

Preparation time: 40 minutes

Nutritional values: Calories-295kcal|Carbs-50g|Protein-50g|Fat-10g

Ingredients

- 1 pkg (142 g) arugula, baby
- 0.68 kg boneless and skinless chicken breasts
- 237 mL broth (chicken or vegetable)
- 1 pkg fresh rosemary, small
- 4 garlic cloves
- Heavy whipped cream (118 mL)

- Parmesan cheese (28 g)
- Penne pasta/spaghetti, 283 g
- 1 can of pure pumpkin purée (398 mL)
- Pepper (black)
- Red pepper flakes
- Olive oil (extra virgin)
- Salt

Directions

1. Fresh produce should be washed and dried. (If the arugula comes pre-washed, skip it.)
2. Load a large pot quarter with warm water (from the water tap), cover, and bring to a simmer over high heat.
3. Transfer 1 cup of Parmesan to a small bowl and finely grate it.
4. Using a moderate flame, heat up a skillet.
5. As the pan warms up, blot the chicken dry using paper towels, then put it on a work surface. Slice the chicken in half uniformly with a knife adjacent to the cutting board to shape thin cutlets. On both sides, sprinkle the cutlets with salt and pepper.
6. When the skillet is wet, drizzle in the olive oil and swirl it around to cover the sides.

7. Cook the chicken cutlets in the pan for 2 to 4 minutes per side, or until lightly browned on the outside and cook through in the middle. Shift to a plate and keep it warm by covering it with foil. If required, cook in batches.
8. Close the pot and sprinkle the water with salt until the water comes to a simmer, then add the pasta and whisk for a few seconds. Cook the pasta for 11 to 12 minutes, uncovered (as per package directions). In a colander, rinse the pasta.
9. Trim and cut the garlic's root ends; slice and mince or squeeze the garlic.
10. Turn down the heat to moderate and incorporate more oil into the pan until the chicken has been shifted.
11. Cook the rosemary sprigs in the skillet for 1 to 2 minutes or until they tend to brown. Leave the oil in the skillet and move to a paper towel-lined pan.
12. After transferring the rosemary, transfer the pumpkin purée, crushed red pepper, and garlic to the pan and cook, constantly stirring, for 1 to 2 minutes, until tangy.
13. In a pan, combine the cream, broth, and Parmesan. Cook, constantly stirring, for 1 to 2 minutes, or until the mix is thoroughly mixed, then turn off the heat.

14. In the same pan, incorporate the pasta and arugula; whisk until the pasta is completely covered with the sauce.
15. Remove the leaves one by one with your hands, keeping a sprig of rosemary at the tip. Remove the sprigs from the fried leaves and cut them; move to a small bowl.
16. Put the chicken on a work surface and cut it into pieces on the diagonal.
17. To eat, divide the pasta among the bowls, top with the chicken pieces, and top with the crispy rosemary leaves. Have fun.

24. POACHED EGGS WITH RED WINE SAUCE

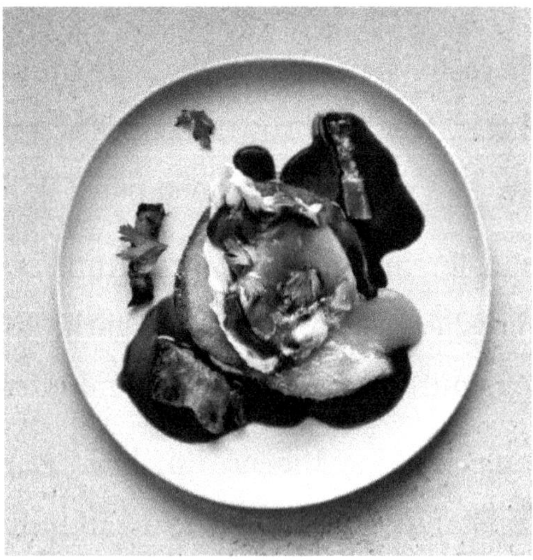

Serving: 8

Preparation time: 1hr 30min

Nutritional values: Calories-436kcal|Carbs-25g|Protein-14g|Fat-23g

Ingredients

- 8 eggs (fresh)
- 1 750 mL bottle of fruity red wine
- 2 cups brown veal/chicken stock (500 ml/16 fl oz.)
- 1 finely sliced onion
- 1 finely chopped carrot
- 1 finely diced celery stalk
- 1 garlic clove, minced,
- Thyme sprigs, parsley leaves, and a bay leaf bouquet garni
- Black peppercorns, 1/2 tsp.
- A pinch of pepper and salt

For Garnish:

- 2 tsp. unsalted butter
- 16 to 20 baby onions, peeled
- 1/4 pound (125 g/4 oz.) mushrooms,
- Cut 1/4 pound (125 g/4 oz.) bacon, chopped.

For The Croutes:

- 8 slices white bread, 1/4 inch thick (6 mm) frying oil

For Thicker Sauce

- 2 tbsp. unsalted butter
- Flour (two tablespoons)

Directions

1. In a wide shallow skillet, take the wine & stock to a rapid boil to poach the eggs. Split four eggs one by one into the simmering liquid, allowing the bubbles to turn the eggs. Reduce the heat to low and poach the eggs for 4 - 5 minutes, or until the yolks are set but still tender. Using a slotted spoon, scrape the eggs and drain on paper towels. Continue to poach the leftover eggs in almost the same manner. Put the eggs aside after pruning the sticky edges with scissors. Simmer the onion, carrot, celery, garlic, bouquet garni, and peppercorns in the poaching liquid for 20 to 25 minutes, or until the liquid is condensed and decreased by half.

2. Meanwhile, prepare the garnish: In a large skillet, melt half the butter, incorporate the mushrooms, then sauté unless tender, around 2 to 3 minutes. Remove the mushrooms and cook the bacon in the remaining butter until it is brown. Drain the bacon on paper towels after extracting it from the skillet. Include the baby onions and cook gently once brown and soft, around 10 to 15 minutes, rotating the pan often to ensure even color.

Drain all of the fat, then substitute the mushrooms & bacon in the pan and put it aside.

3. Using a circular or oval cutter, slice the bread into 8 shapes slightly larger than a poached egg for the croûtes. In a frying pan, warm 1/4 inch (6 mm) of oil over medium heat. Cook the croûtes in batches until golden brown on both sides, around 1 to 2 minutes each side. Using paper towels, absorb extra moisture. Set aside the croûtes.

4. To stiffen the sauce, smash the butter with a fork on a plate and whisk in the flour until a soft paste develops. Whisk a piece of the kneaded butter into the boiling wine mixture at a time before the mixture thickens sufficiently to easily cover a spoon. Grate the sauce over the mushrooms, baby onions, & bacon garnish, lowering on the carrot, onion, and celery to absorb as much liquid and flavor as possible. Get the sauce to a simmer, then test and season to taste.

5. To cook ahead of time, poach the eggs in a bowl of cool water in the refrigerator for up to a day. Refrigerate the sauce as well as the garnishes. If the croûtes are tightly sealed and heated in a low oven, they will be perfect.

6. Reheat the eggs for serving by soaking them in warm water for at least a minute. Braise the garnish & sauce on the stovetop if possible, and steam the croûtes in the

oven. Place the croûtes on hot plates to serve. Sap the eggs on paper towels, put one on each croûte, and then spoon over the sauce & garnish.

25. VEGAN LASAGNA WITH SPINACH AND RICOTTA

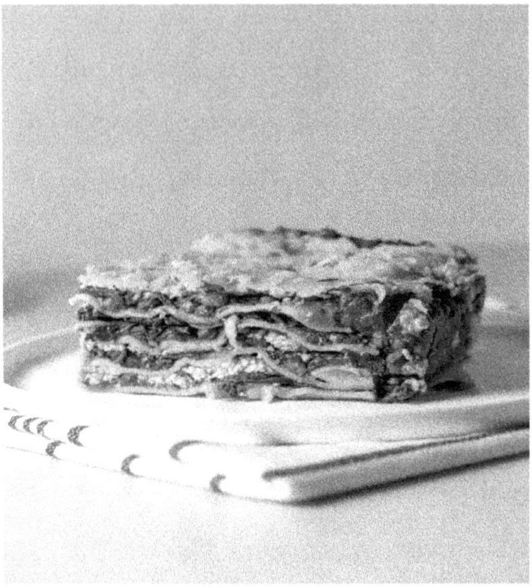

Serving: 6

Preparation time: 1hr 15min

Nutritional values: Calories-516kcal|Carbs-72g|Protein-22g|Fat-20g

Ingredients

- San Marzano Tomato Sauce, 4.25 cup
- 6 cups spinach (baby)
- 1 pound sliced mushrooms or canned artichoke hearts)
- A half onion, finely chopped.

- No-boil lentil lasagna noodles (12 oz.)
- OPTIONAL: 6-ounce vegan smoked Gouda cheese slices
- 1 large sliced heirloom tomato
- Basil leaves (about 1/3 cup) (for garnish)
- 1 pinch flakes red pepper

For Cashew Ricotta Cheese:

- 2 cups cashews, fresh
- 3/4 cup of water
- 1 lemon, freshly squeezed
- 2 garlic cloves, grated
- 1/2 tsp. of onion powder
- A half teaspoon of garlic powder
- 1/2 teaspoon salt

Directions

1. Make the tomato sauce ahead of time.
2. To make the cashew ricotta, follow these steps:
3. Rinse the cashews and soak them in hot water for 20 minutes. Drain and rinse them again, then combine them with the rest of the ingredients in an efficient blender (or food processor). Process until the mixture is

creamy as well as smooth. Put it in the fridge until prepared to be using.

4. Preheat the oven to 400 degrees Fahrenheit.
5. Preheat a large saucepan over medium heat. Sauté the onion with a bit of salt in a splash of water until opaque, around 5 minutes. Cook for another ten min or so until the mushrooms are wilted and the moisture has evaporated. Mix with sea salt to taste. Keep it aside until you need it.
6. Bring another tsp. of water and the spinach to the same skillet. Season with a sprinkle of sea salt after sautéing until wilted. Drain the water in a colander. When the liquid is cold enough to manage, squeeze as far as you can out of it with your hands. Place aside.
7. Prepare the lasagna pan (an 8X12 pan would suffice) by putting 1.5 cups of tomato sauce in the bottom. Layer sufficiently lasagna noodles to reach the bottom and partially overlap each other. Depending on the form of your pan, you can need to crack a few of them to fill up any holes on the edges.
8. Spread the cashew ricotta over all the bottom in an even layer. (If desired, add a dash of freshly crushed nutmeg at this point.)

9. The toasted spinach & mushrooms go on top, accompanied by 1.25 cup tomato sauce.
10. Finish with a sheet of the leftover sauce and another layer of lasagna noodles, partially overlapping each other.
11. Coating with a layer of vegan smoked Gouda and slices of heirloom tomatoes on top. Season with a pinch of red pepper flakes and a sprinkle of sea salt.
12. Top the lasagna tray with aluminum foil (or a lid) and bake for 45 to 50 minutes or until the noodles are cooked.
13. Allow 15 minutes for cooling and setting while serving with fresh basil on top.

26. HAM AND ASPARAGUS OMELET WITH PARSLEY AND POTATOES

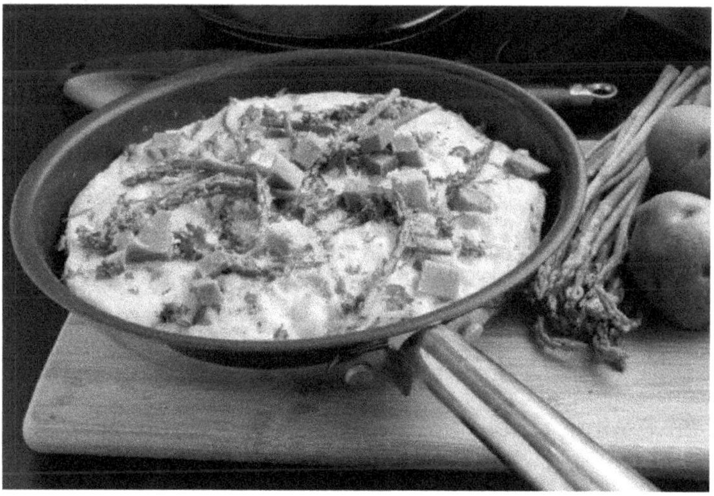

Serving: 2

Preparation time: 50 minutes

Nutritional values: Calories-288kcal|Carbs-15g|Protein-19g|Fat-16g

Ingredients

- Fresh potatoes, 7 oz.
- Salt to taste
- White asparagus, 5 oz.
- One onion
- Prosciutto, 2 oz.
- 2 parsley sprigs
- Three eggs
- 1 tbsp. oil (vegetable)
- Peppers

Directions

1. Wash the potatoes thoroughly. Cook unless potatoes are tender in a pan of heating salted water, around 20 minutes, then extract and cool. Shave the outer sheath of asparagus stalks, then cut the woody ends once the potatoes are boiling. Cook the asparagus for 15 minutes in boiling salted water unless soft, then drain well and cool. Peel and finely cut the onion.

2. Cut the asparagus & potatoes into tiny pieces.
3. Slice the prosciutto into segments.
4. Wash the parsley by rinsing it, shaking it out, plucking the leaves, and chopping them finely. In a mixing bowl, whisk together the eggs and minced parsley.
5. In a nonstick pan, heat the oil over moderate flame. Cook, constantly stirring, until onions are translucent, around 1-2 minutes.
6. Cook for 2 minutes, or until potatoes are cooked through.
7. Cook for 1 minute, or until asparagus is cooked through.
8. Season with salt, then pepper, and add the prosciutto.
9. Incorporate the eggs into the pan, cover, and cook on low heat for 5-6 minutes, or until set. Remove from the pan and serve right away.

27. Raw Rainbow Collard Green wraps with Curry Sunflower seeds

Serving: 4

Preparation time: 30 minutes

Nutritional values: Calories-113kcal|Carbs-14g|Protein-5g|Fat-5g

Ingredients

- 1 cup soaked raw sunflower seeds

- 1/2 cup chopped celery (approximately 2 - 2.5 stalks)
- 1/2 cup carrots, shredded
- 1/2 cup cilantro herbs, packed
- 1/3 cup roughly chopped green onion
- 1/3 cup of diced bell pepper
- Half cup of raisins (optional)
- 3 tablespoons tahini
- 1 tbsp. extra virgin olive oil
- 1 tablespoon of water
- 1.5 tbsp. lemon juice (approximately 1/2 lemon)
- Apple cider vinegar, 2 teaspoons
- 1.5 teaspoon curry powder
- 1 tsp. turmeric powder
- Half teaspoon of salt
- Sprinklings of freshly crushed pepper
- 5 to 6 collard leaves for the wraps
- Cabbage, carrots, cucumber, avocado, fresh basil, mango, and all other fillings you like

Directions

1. In a food processor, mix all of the ingredients mentioned

under the sunflower seed mixture. Mix before the optimal quality is achieved.

2. Set aside whatever other vegetables you'll be using for the wraps.
3. Chop the collard green stem ends off for the collard wraps. Bring a pot of water to a near-boiling point, then chop up the leaves for 10 seconds before scraping them with tongs from the hot pot. The leaves are more pliable after being blanched.
4. **Assemble the parts and roll them out:** The seed mixture can be spread around the center of the leaves. Toss in some vegetables on top. Fold the right & left sides in, then fold the nearest side up. Roll away from you as tightly as possible.
5. Round it in half and serve it! The seed mixture can keep in the fridge for 5 days.

28. ROASTED CHICKEN BREASTS WITH WALNUTS, DATES & OLIVES

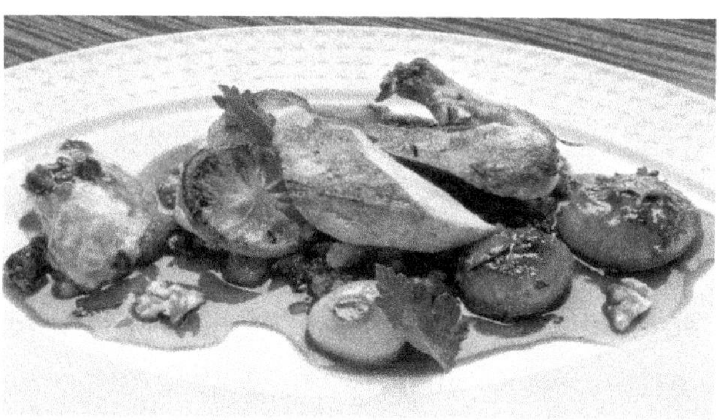

Serving: 6

Preparation: 1hr 35min

Nutritional values: Calories-403kcal|Carbs-19g|Protein-30g|Fat-23g

Ingredients

- Six boneless breasts of chicken, halves
- 5 to 6 Medjool dates, charred and chopped
- 2/3 cup of red wine vinegar
- 2 tbsp. extra virgin olive oil
- 3/4 cup of toasted walnut pieces of California
- 1/3 cup pitted and diced nicoise or kalamata olives
- 3/4 cup chicken stock, concentrated
- 1 and a half tbsp. butter
- 3 tbsp. Italian parsley, finely chopped

Directions

1. In a small bowl, mix the dates & vinegar and set aside for an hour or two. Set the oven to 325 degrees Fahrenheit. In a wide ovenproof skillet, heat the olive oil over a moderate flame, then bring the chicken until brown for 2 minutes across each side. Put the pan in the oven for 12–14 min, or until the chicken is completely cooked. Place the chicken on a serving platter and serve

2. Put the walnuts, olives, as well as stock in a skillet over a high flame, along with the stored dates & vinegar. Boil for a few seconds, scratching the bottom of the pan with a slotted spoon to pick up some flavorful pieces. Stir in the butter and parsley before the butter has melted. Season with salt and pepper as required, then spill over the chicken & serve right away.
3. Onion Walnut & Pancetta Topping can be added as a garnish if needed.

29. BUCKWHEAT AND BEAN SOUP

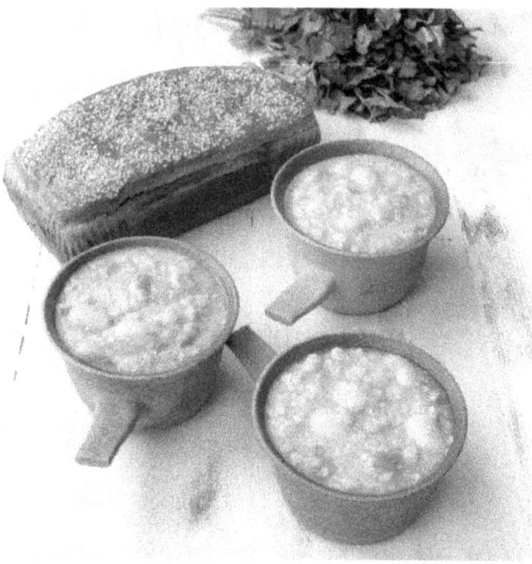

Serving: 12

Preparation time: 3hr 30min

Nutritional values: Calories-164kcal|Carbs-30g|Protein-7g|Fat-3.2g

Ingredients

- 5-6 bones / 800 g marrow bones (you may also use frozen bones)
- 300 g buckwheat (if you're not gluten-free, you can substitute pearl barley)
- 500 grams split peas/yellow lentils (also called Chana dal)
- 1 finely diced onion (peeled)
- Peeled and finely diced 5 carrots (approx. 700g)
- 2 celery stalks, chopped finely
- 9 pints iced water
- Sugar, 3 tsp.
- 2 tbsp. Herbamare or 2 cubes of chicken/vegetable stock
- 4 tins 400 g canned butterbeans, soaked and rinsed, sea salt or pink salt white pepper Himalayan salt

Directions

1. In different bowls, soak the buckwheat as well as yellow lentils for 40 minutes in cold water.
2. Organize the marrow bones in the bottom of a wide (apx.7 liters volume) stockpot, surround with 9 pints of ice water, then take to a boil and simmer for 30-40 min, trawling away any dirt that rises to the surface along the

way – you can reduce the heat to a low simmer when skimming, but you must leave the water boiling for the most part.

3. Season with sea salt and a pinch of white pepper after the boiling period is up, and you've skimmed off as much dirt as practicable from the top, then introduce the sugar as well as Herbamare (or stock cubes) and taste.
4. Wash the soaked buckwheat in cool, flowing water until the water runs smooth, drain well, and put in a clean bowl. Then, along with the celery, onions, and carrots, add the yellow lentils & buckwheat to the pot.
5. Take the pot back to a simmer, then reduce to low heat and simmer for 2 1/2 hours, stirring periodically to keep some of the ingredients from sticking to the bottom of the pan.
6. Turn off the heat under the pan and set aside for 15 minutes before scraping the bones and setting aside for another 30 minutes before eating.
7. Present with some crusty, fresh bread for dipping.

30. MUSTARD – ORANGE-GLAZED PORK CHOP

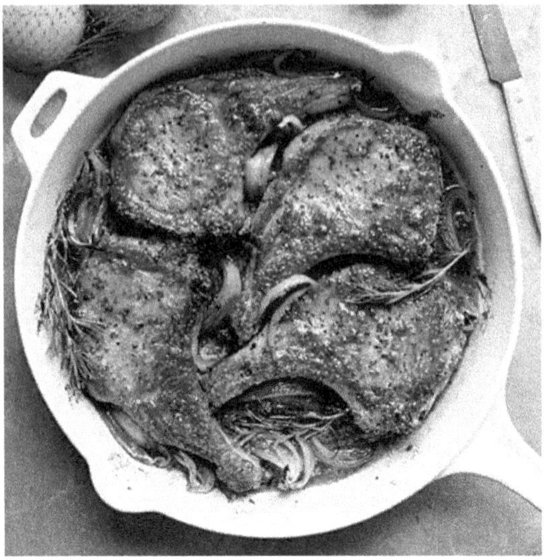

Serving: 4

Preparation time: 40 minutes

Nutritional values: Calories-303kcal|Carbs-14g|Protein-28g|Fat-10g

Ingredients

- 1/2 cup orange juice, freshly squeezed (about 2 oranges)
- 2 tbsp. marmalade of orange
- 1 tbsp. mustard (whole grain)
- 1 tbsp. oil of canola
- Pork loin chops, bone-in, 6 oz. (1 inch thick)
- Kosher salt (1/4 teaspoon)
- 1/4 teaspoon. Black pepper, freshly ground

- 2 sprigs of rosemary
- 1/2-inch wedges of 1 red onion, medium-sized
- Lime juice, 2 tbsp.

Directions

1. Preheat the oven to 425 degrees Fahrenheit.
2. In a pan over medium heat, mix the juice, marmalade, and mustard. Bring to a simmer, then reduce to low heat and cook for 15 minutes, or until the mixture has thickened into a syrup.
3. On medium-high heat, preheat a wide ovenproof skillet. Swirl in the oil to evenly cover around. Add salt and pepper to the pork. Cook for 5 minutes, or until browned, in the skillet. Place the pork in the pan and add the rosemary and onion. Spill the juice solution over the pork and bake for ten min at 425°F, unless a thermometer measures 140°F. On a plate, arrange the onion and rosemary. Return the pan to a high heat state and add the lime juice. Cook for another 4 minutes, or until the liquid has thickened to a syrupy consistency. Drizzle sauce over pork on a platter.

31. MISO - COD SKEWERS WITH GREENS

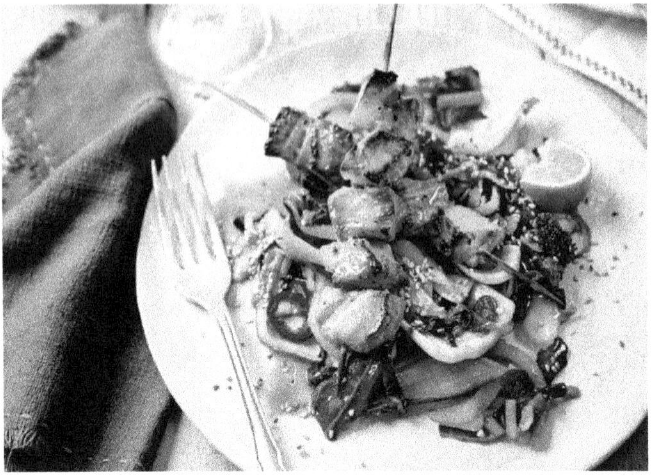

Serving: 2

Preparation time: 30 minutes

Nutritional values: Calories-382kcal|Carbs-31g|Protein-37g|Fat-12g

Ingredients

- Cod fillets, Skinless, sliced into cubes, 340g pack
- Sesame seeds, 1 tbsp.
- 220g veggies stir-fry medley in a pack
- Sesame oil (1 tbsp.)
- Pak Choi (250g pack)
- 1 tablespoon of hoisin sauce
- 1 tablespoon of sweet chili sauce

For the Marinade

- 1 tablespoon of miso paste
- Agave nectar, 2 tablespoons
- 1 tablespoon mirin
- 2 tbsp. soy sauce (light)
- 1/2 lime wedges, juiced, with extras to serve

Directions

1. In a bowl, mix all of the ingredients for the marinade; season with a pinch of black pepper. Cover and let it cool for at least 15 minutes or overnight after adding the fish.
2. Heat up the grill to an elevated temp. Cook up the sesame seeds in a small dry frying pan until golden. Place in a safe place until required.
3. Using skewers, thread the fish into a foil-lined sheet pan. Drizzle any residual marinade over the top. Cook for 2-3 minutes on either hand or until cooked through and finely charred.
4. Meanwhile, reserve the seed and finely sliced chili from the stir-fry pack for garnish.
5. In a wide frying pan, heat the sesame oil over high heat. Stir-fry for 4 minutes, or until the vegetables (except the chili) are just soft, with the hoisin & sweet chili sauces. Sprinkle the sesame seeds and chili over the top. Serve

with additional lime wedges for pressing over the fish skewers.

32. COFFEE RUBBED BURGERS

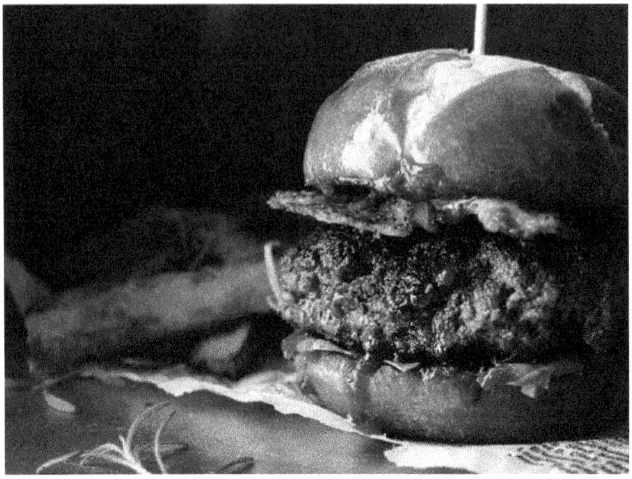

Serving: 4

Preparation time: 40 minutes

Nutritional values: Calories-471kcal|Carbs-17.2g|Protein-42g|Fat-24g

Ingredients

Seasoning for Coffee Rub:

- 1 tbsp. Coffee (ground)
- 1/2 tablespoon. Salt
- 2 tsp. paprika (smoked)
- 1 tsp. onion powder
- 2 tsp. brown sugar

- 1 tsp. crushed garlic
- 1/2 teaspoon cayenne pepper
- A half tsp. of coriander
- A half tsp. of oregano
- 1/4 teaspoon black pepper

For Burgers:

- 1 pound of ground beef
- 4 smoked Gouda cheese slices
- 1 onion, cut thickly into rings
- Pretzel rolls

For Homemade BBQ Sauce:

- 1 cup ketchup (organic)
- 1/4 cup of apple cider vinegar
- 1/2 cup water
- 3 tbsp. Brown Sugar
- 1 tbsp. Onion Powder
- 1/2 tsp. Worcestershire sauce
- 1 tsp. yellow mustard
- 1/2 teaspoon freshly squeezed lemon juice
- Garlic Powder (1/2 teaspoon)

- 1 tsp. paprika (smoked)
- A half teaspoon of butter

Directions

1. In a small bowl, mix all of the ingredients for the coffee rub.
2. With the use of a patty press, if you have one, gently shape four patties. The spice rub can be applied across both parts of the patties. There is plenty for the four of them. Using your fingertips, gently brush the spices onto the patties.
3. When the grill is heating up, place the patties on a wire rack in the fridge for 30 minutes to allow for airflow. This is an important step that cannot be skipped.
4. Cut the onions into thicker rings and spray them with olive oil or Italian seasoning without splitting them apart.
5. Heat up the grill to high and cook the burgers over direct heat for a few minutes (based on thickness). Cook for a couple of minutes, on the other hand. Reduce the heat to low and simmer until the chicken is cooked to your preference. Pieces of cheese can be put on top and melted right before serving.

6. Put the onions on the supplementary side of the grill on low heat at the same time. When you see marks on the grill and the onions starting to soften, flip them.
7. Pretzel buns can be grilled for a few minutes unless light brown.
8. Top the burger with the onion & bbq sauce on the pretzel bun.

For the Barbeque Sauce:

1. In a wide skillet over medium heat, mix the first 7 ingredients. To combine, mix or stir all together. Get the spices to a simmer, stirring constantly.
2. Reduce heat to low and cook for thirty min, stirring frequently.
3. Add the cold butter and blend properly. Cook for another five min to thicken.

33. MATCHA GREEN TEA ICE CREAM

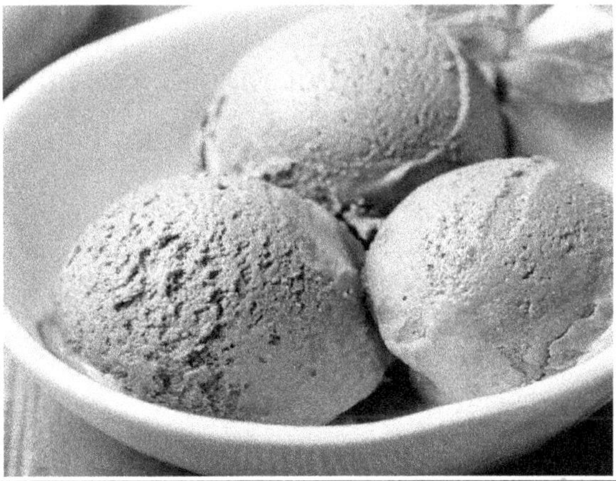

Serving: 8

Preparation time: 5hr 5min

Nutritional values: Calories-319kcal|Carbs-22g|Protein-4g|Fat-24.3g

Ingredients

- 1 tbsp. matcha green tea powder (or more, depending on personal choice)
- 1 cup of whole milk
- Heavy whipped cream, 2 cup
- ¾ cup of white sugar
- Two eggs

Directions

1. In a bowl, stir matcha powder to eliminate any lumps; incorporate a dash of milk and stir until absolutely dissolved. Whisk the leftover milk into the matcha mixture gradually.
2. In a medium-low-heat pan, mix cream and matcha mixture; cook, stirring periodically until cooked through, around 5 minutes.
3. In a mixing bowl, combine the sugar and eggs. Pour 1/2 cup of the hot matcha mixture into the egg mixture and

stir well. Repeat for the remainder of the matcha mixture. Transfer the mixture to the pot.

4. On medium-low heat, cook and whisk the matcha mixture until it is thoroughly cooked, around 3 minutes. Remove the pan from the heat and allow it to cool at room temperature. Refrigerate for at least 4 hours before serving.
5. Load an ice cream maker halfway with the chilled matcha mixture and freeze as per the manufacturer's directions.

34. AVOCADO WRAP WITH CHICKPEAS

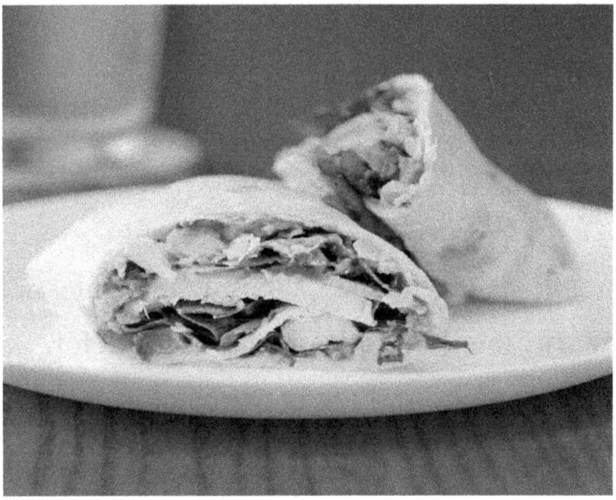

Serving: 2

Preparation time: 25 minutes

Nutritional values: Calories-315kcal|Carbs-38g|Protein-6g|Fat-18g

Ingredients

- Chickpeas, 1 can (240g or 1.5 cups)
- 1 tablespoon of maple syrup
- 1 teaspoon cumin
- Turmeric, 1 teaspoon
- 1 teaspoon salt to render the avocado sauce
- 1 avocado, peeled and mashed
- 1/2 cup minced fresh dill
- 2 tablespoons tamari
- Lemon juice (1/2 lemon)
- 3 tbsp. yogurt (soy)
- 2 gluten-free tortillas, large

Directions

1. In a nonstick frying pan, combine the chickpeas, cumin, turmeric, maple syrup, and salt, & cook for 5-6 minutes, thinning out around 1/2 of the chickpeas.
2. Meanwhile, make the avocado sauce by combining the mashed avocado, lemon juice, fresh dill and tamari, and also soy yogurt in a mixing bowl.
3. Assemble the wrap until the chickpeas are ready. Spread a coating of avocado sauce on top, then top with chickpeas. Complete the process. Before turning up the

bottom edge, pull over the sides. Serve right away or keep refrigerated for 3-4 days.

35. QUINOA KALE STUFFING WITH SQUASH RINGS

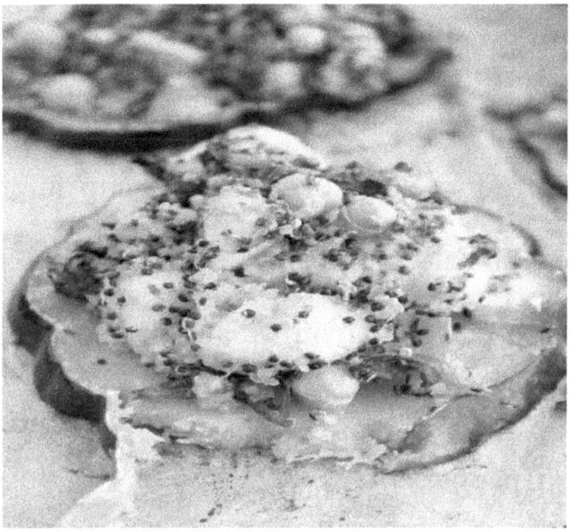

Serving: 10

Preparation time: 40 minutes

Nutritional values: Calories-119kcal|Carbs-18g|Protein-4g|Fat-3g

Ingredients

- 1 acorn squash, washed & thinly diced uniformly into 1/8 inch thick slices with the seeds extracted
- 1 pinch of salt
- 1 pinch of pepper
- 1 tbsp. extra virgin olive oil

For Stuffing of Quinoa:

- 1 tsp. extra virgin olive oil
- 2 finely diced tiny shallots
- 1/3 cup sweet bell pepper, diced
- 1 peeled sweet potato, cut into 1/2 inch pieces
- 2/3 cup quinoa (uncooked) or 1 1/4 cup quinoa (cooked)
- 1 cup fresh kale, chopped
- Chickpeas, 2/3 cup (canned and drained, or cooked)
- Salt (1/4 teaspoon)
- 1/4 tsp. pepper
- 1 tablespoon finely grated oregano (or 1 tsp. of dried oregano)
- 1/4 cup Parmesan cheese, grated (ignore if vegan)

Directions

1. Preheat oven to 425 degrees Fahrenheit.
2. In a large pan, sauté the shallots & bell peppers along with the olive oil over medium heat to make the stuffing.
3. Integrate the sweet potatoes and quinoa into the mix (if raw, otherwise if using cooked quinoa, bring it in later).

4. If using fresh quinoa, add 1 cup of warm water to the sweet potato mixture; if using prepared quinoa, transfer just half a cup of hot water to the sweet potato mixture.
5. Reduce the heat to a lower level and cover the pot for around 15 minutes, or until the sweet potatoes are soft and the quinoa is cooked (if using raw).
6. Remove the lid from the pot and check for any residual water at the bottom. If there is some water, leave the lid uncovered and cook on lower for another 2 minutes, or until the water has vanished. Toss in the quinoa for a few seconds at this stage.
7. Add the kale, chickpeas, parmesan cheese, seasoning, and oregano to the quinoa sweet potato mixture when it's finished. Put aside after a thorough tossing.
8. Place the squash rings on a parchment-lined baking sheet and season with salt, pepper, and olive oil.
9. Place around half a cup of the prepared stuffing on top of each squash ring. Stuff the rings with stuffing in the center and on the edges, leaving a small border.
10. Preheat the oven to 350°F and bake the baking sheet for 15-18 minutes, or unless the squash is fork-ready.

36. APPLE PECAN ARUGULA SALAD

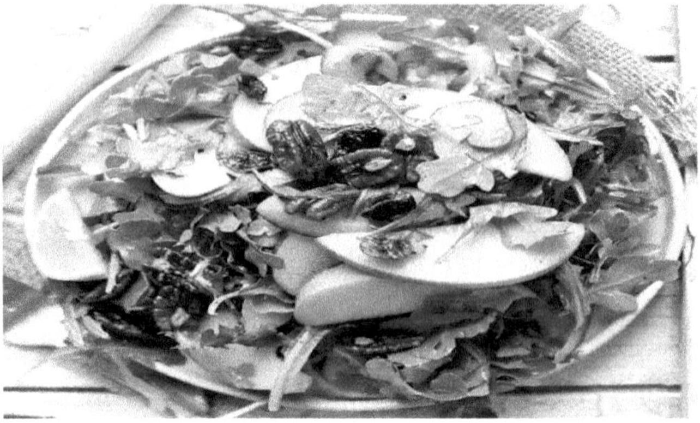

Serving: 4

Preparation time: 15 minutes

Nutritional values: Calories-258kcal|Carbs-21g|Protein-3f|Fat-20g

Ingredients

- 1/2 cup pecans, raw
- Arugula, 7 oz. (organic when possible)
- 2 tiny apples, peeled, cut into quarters, cored, and sliced thinly lengthwise (1 tart, 1 sweet)
- 1/4 onion, red (thinly sliced)
- 2 tablespoons cranberries, dried (optional)

For Dressing

- 1 large lemon, squeezed (1 lemon contains 3 tablespoons or 45 milliliters)

- 1 tablespoon of maple syrup
- 1 pinch each of sea salt and black pepper
- 3 tablespoons extra virgin olive oil

Directions

1. Preheat the oven to 350°F (176°C) and spread pecans out on a baking sheet.
2. Bake pecans for around 8-10 minutes, or until aromatic and rich golden brown. Remove the pot from the oven and put it aside.
3. As the pecans toast, prepare the remainder of the salad ingredients and mix them in a large mixing bowl.
4. To make the dressing, combine certain ingredients in a mixing bowl and whisk or shake vigorously to combine. Taste and make the required changes to the taste.
5. Toss the salad with the pecans and the dressing. Toss to mix and serve straight away.
6. Refrigerate leftovers (dressing apart from salad) for 2-3 days, wrapped (though perfect when fresh). When properly wrapped, the dressing can last for 2-3 days at room temperature.

37. WARM CHICKEN AND CHICORY SALAD

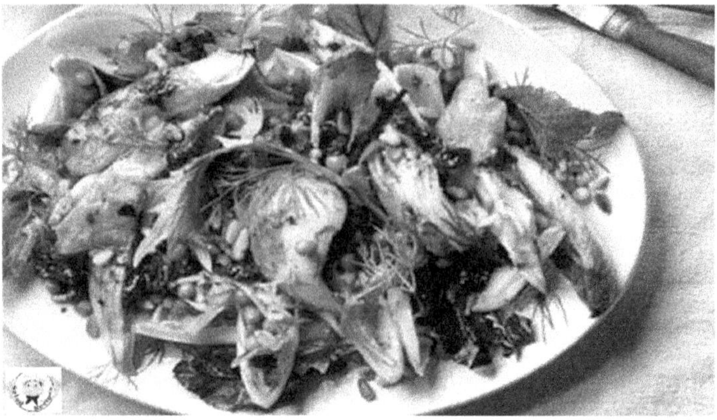

Serving: 4-6

Preparation time: 2hr 30min

Nutritional values: Calories-765kcal|Carbs-17g|Protein-58g|Fat-52g

Ingredients

- Whole chicken, 1.6 kg
- 4 tbsp. room temperature butter
- 1 tbsp. sherry vinegar plus 200ml
- 200g peas, frozen
- 3 tbsp. extra virgin olive oil
- 1/2 teaspoon caster sugar
- 50 grams of raisins
- 15g dill pack, finely chopped

- 3 heads chicory, orange, red, or a hybrid of the two
- 50g salad leaves, mixed (rocket & chard mix)
- 100g toasted pine nut
- Serve with crusty bread

Directions

1. Preheat oven to 160 degrees Celsius/140 degrees Celsius fan/gas 3. Butter the both in and out of chicken and season it well. Place it in a tiny roasting pan, cover it with foil, and spill the Sherry vinegar over it. Cook for 2 hours.
2. In the meantime, prepare the remaining ingredients. Cook the peas for 1 minute, or until they are just soft. Drain well, then easily cool in cold water while draining and setting aside.
3. Remove the chicken from the oven after it has cooked for 2 hours. Increase the oven temperature to 220C/200C fan/gas 7 and pour the liquids into a jug. Cook for another 20-30 minutes (uncovered) unless golden.
4. Scrape the fat from the liquids, then simmer until the juices are reduced to around 100ml. Taste, then add the remaining tablespoon of vinegar, olive oil, and caster sugar, along with the raisins, to your serving bowl.
5. After the chicken has completed its second roasting, set it aside until it is cold enough to touch (or put on a pair

of clean plastic gloves), then cut the meat from the carcass into larger chunks and place it on the serving dish. Toss together the dill, chicory, lettuce leaves, pine nuts, and peas with your hands. With crusty bread, serve right away.

38. COCONUT, CHICKEN, AND KALE CURRY

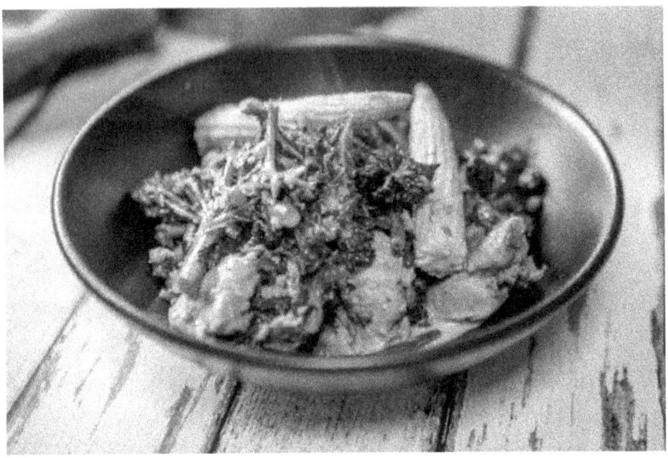

Serving: 4

Preparation time: 45 minutes

Nutritional values: Calories-451kcal|Carbs-31g|Protein-42g|Fat19g

Ingredients

- 1 tablespoon of groundnut oil
- 1 diced onion
- 1 seeded and minced green chili
- 2 chopped or crushed garlic cloves

- 15 g grated or chopped fresh ginger
- 100g thawed green lentils (optional soaking)
- 2 tablespoons curry powder (medium)
- 2 anise star
- 250 milliliters chicken broth
- 250 milliliters coconut milk
- 1 1/2 tablespoon lime juice
- Sultanas, 50g
- 490g of chicken breast, cubed to 2.5cm
- Broccoli tender stem, 200g
- 100g cut and halved green beans
- 100 grams of baby corn
- 2 handfuls of kale, sliced

Directions

1. In a saucepan, add the oil over low heat. Fry for 5 minutes with the onion, chili, garlic, and ginger.
2. Stir in the lentils, curry powder, and star anise until well mixed. Put in the chicken broth and simmer for 10 minutes, or until it has been decreased by half.
3. Add the coconut milk, lemon juice, and sultanas to the curry, then put the chicken chunks and cook for 15

minutes. Cook for about 10 minutes with broccoli, green beans, kale, and baby corn until the chicken is cooked through and no pink meat remains. Take out the star anise, then serve right away.

39. Puffed buckwheat toasted muesli

Serving: 10

Preparation time: 35 minutes

Nutritional values: Calories-211kcal|Carbs-19g|Protein-4g|Fat-14g

Ingredients

- 2 cups buckwheat puffed
- 1 cup oats, rolled
- Flakes of coconut (1/2 cup)
- Seeds of coconut (about 1/3 cup)
- Sunflower seeds, 1/3 cup
- 1/3 cup cashews, chopped
- 2 tsp. cinnamon powder (optional)
- 1/3 cup liquid sweetener (maple syrup, honey, or some other liquid sweetener)
- 2 teaspoon vanilla extract – Optional
- 1/4 cup coconut oil melted

Directions

1. Preheat the oven to 150 degrees Celsius (300 degrees Fahrenheit) and cover a wide baking tray with parchment paper.
2. Integrate the buckwheat, coconut flakes, nuts, oats, seeds, and cinnamon in a wide mixing bowl.
3. Melt the coconut oil, maple syrup, and vanilla together until smooth and runny, whisking constantly. (This may be done on the stovetop or in the microwave.) Bring the liquid over the dried mixture and stir vigorously to cover all of the dry ingredients.
4. Using a spatula, uniformly distribute the mixture around the baking sheet. To avoid burns across the edges, bake for 20-25 minutes, swirling the mixture gently a few times. Remove the tray from the oven and set it aside to cool completely; the muesli may crisp up while it cools.
5. It could last 2 to 3 weeks if kept in an airtight jar.

40. BROCCOLI AND GREEN KALE SOUP

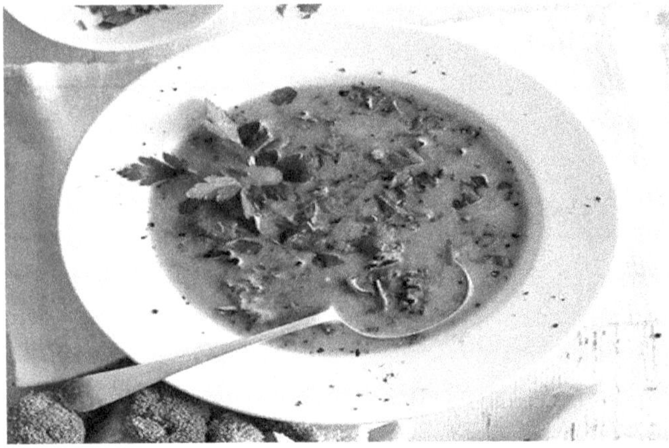

Serving: 2

Preparation time: 20 minutes

Nutritional values: Calories-182kcal|Carbs-14g|Protein-10g|Fat-8g

Ingredients

- 500ml stock, prepared in a jug with one tablespoon bouillon powder & boiling water
- 1 tablespoon of sunflower oil
- 3cm/1in piece fresh turmeric root, stripped and diced, or ½ teaspoon ground turmeric
- Pinch of pink Himalayan salt
- 2 garlic cloves, sliced
- Thumb-sized piece ginger, sliced

- 1/2 teaspoon ground coriander
- 85g broccoli 200g courgettes, finely cut
- 100g chopped kale
- 1 lime, zested and juiced
- Small pack parsley, finely chopped, with a few fresh leaves saved for serving

Directions

1. In a deep skillet, heat the oil, then add the garlic, coriander, ginger, turmeric, and salt. Cook for 2 minutes on moderate flame, then add 3 tablespoon water to give the spices a little more moisture.
2. Stir in the courgettes, make sure they are properly coated in all of the spices, then cook for another 3 minutes. Boil for 3 minutes after adding 400ml stock.
3. Integrate the broccoli, kale, and lime juice with the remaining stock in a large mixing bowl. Cook for another 3-4 minutes, or until all of the vegetables are tender.
4. Remove the pan from the heat and stir in the chopped parsley. Blend all together in a high-powered blender until smooth. It'll be pretty green with dark flecks spattered throughout (which is the kale). Lime zest & parsley are additional garnishes.

41. LENTIL AND VEGETABLE SOUP

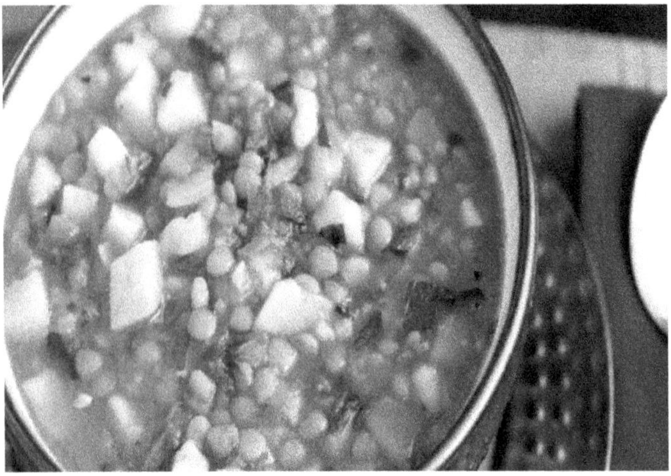

Serving: 10

Preparation time: 45 minutes

Nutritional values: Calories-304kcal|Carbs-51g|Protein-16g|Fat-5g

Ingredients

- 2 cups rinsed dried lentils
- 1 cup rinsed dried quinoa
- 2 shredded carrots
- 1 sweet potato, peeled and cut into small chunks
- 1 chopped yellow onion
- 2 garlic cloves, peeled and minced
- 5 cups low-sodium vegetable broth (no sugar added)

- 4 ounces green chilies, diced
- 2 tsp. chili powder
- 1 tsp. cumin powder
- 1/4 teaspoon red pepper flakes, crushed
- 1 teaspoon freshly ground black pepper
- A half teaspoon of salt (more to taste)
- 2 cups ripped and packed chard, with middle stem cut
- 1 avocado, diced
- 1/2 cup diced fresh cilantro

Directions

1. In a large pot, combine all ingredients except the last three (chard, avocado, and cilantro). Bring to a simmer, then minimize to low heat and cover with a slightly ajar lid.
2. Cook for 30 minutes, or until lentils & quinoa are tender.
3. Cook until the Swiss card has wilted, around 5 minutes.
4. Serve with minced cilantro and sliced avocado on top.

42. TURMERIC ROASTED CRISPY POTATOES

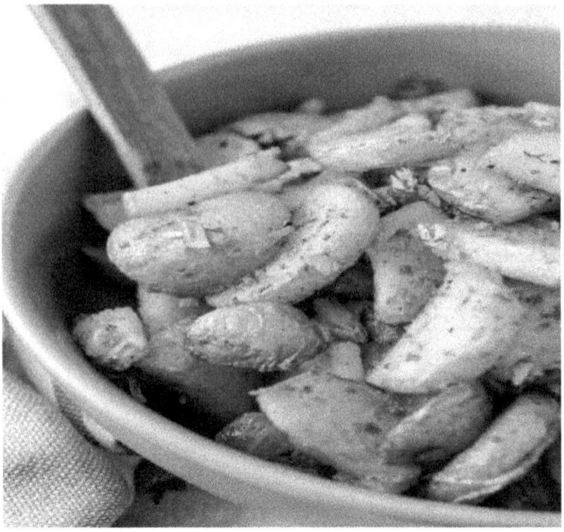

Serving: 6

Preparation time: 35 minutes

Nutritional values: Calories-171kcal|Carbs-25g|Protein-3g|Fat-7g

Ingredients

- 1 minced yellow onion
- 4 garlic cloves, diced or chopped
- 1/2 tbsp. turmeric powder
- 5 cups potatoes
- 1/2 tsp. black pepper
- 1 tsp. salt
- 1/2 tsp. curry powder (optional)

- 3–4 tbsp. extra virgin olive oil

Directions

1. Preheat the oven to 375 degrees Fahrenheit.
2. Using parchment paper, cover a baking dish.
3. Integrate onion, potatoes, garlic, spices, and olive oil in a large Ziploc bag or wide mixing bowl. Toss the potatoes in the mixture until they are evenly covered.
4. Cover the baking sheet halfway with potatoes.
5. Bake for about 30 to 35 min, stirring and tossing the potatoes every ten minutes to ensure even baking.

43. SHAKSHUKA

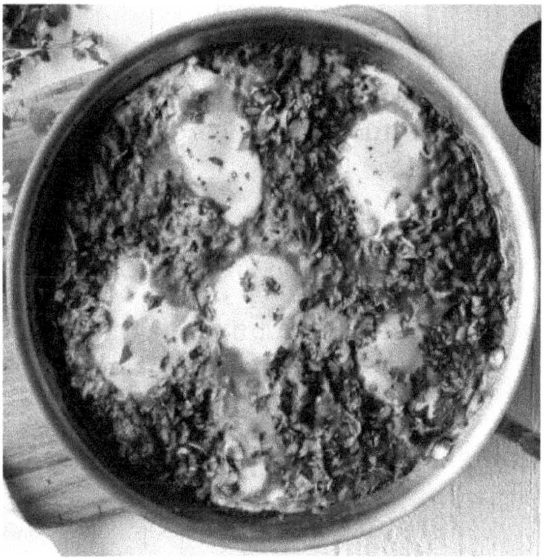

Serving: 6

Preparation time: 30 minutes

Nutritional values: Calories-122kcal|Carbs-10g|Protein-8g|Fat-5g

Ingredients

- 1 medium diced onion
- 1 seeded and sliced red bell pepper
- 4 thinly chopped garlic cloves
- Paprika, 2 tsp.
- 1 teaspoon cumin
- 1/4 tsp. chili powder
- 1 whole peeled 28-ounce can of tomatoes
- 6 large eggs, seasoned to taste with salt and pepper
- 1 tiny bunch chopped fresh cilantro
- 1 tiny bunch of finely chopped parsley

Directions

1. In a wide sauté pan over medium heat, heat the olive oil. Cook for 5 minutes, or until the onion is translucent, before adding the diced bell pepper and onion.
2. Cook for another minute after adding the garlic and spices.
3. Pour the tomatoes & juice into the bowl and use a large spoon to break down the tomatoes. Season with salt and pepper, then reduce to low heat.

4. Make little wells in the sauce with your large spoon and smash the eggs into each well. Cook, covered, for 5 to 8 minutes, or unless the eggs are cooked to your taste.
5. Garnish with cilantro and parsley, if desired.

44. CHOCOLATE AND COCONUT VEGAN ENERGY BALLS

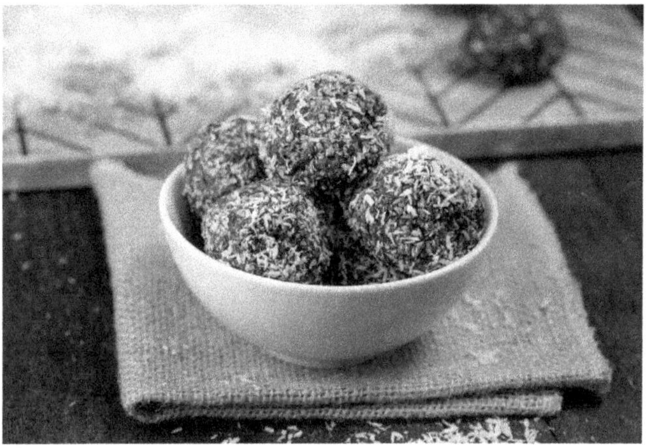

Serving: 22

Preparation time: 20 minutes

Nutritional values: Calories-59kcal|Carbs-6g|Protein-2g|Fat-4g

Ingredients

- Chopped or slivered almonds - 3/4 cup
- 1/2 cup cocoa, unsweetened
- 2 tbsp. flaxseed, ground
- 1/4 teaspoon salt, ground

- 1 1/3 cup organic old-fashioned rolled oats (gluten-free optional)
- Medjool dates, pits separated, 1 pound 16 ounces (if dates are not tender, soak them in water for 20 min first)
- 1/4 cup molten unrefined coconut oil
- 1/4 cup unsweetened coconut, finely shredded

Directions

1. In a food processor, pulse the almond slices for 20-30 seconds or until finely minced.
2. Combine the chocolate, flaxseed, sea salt, and oats in a mixing bowl. Blend for the next 20 seconds or so, once smooth.
3. Integrate the dates with coconut oil in a bowl. Process for 2-3 minutes, or until thoroughly combined. Notice that, based on how sharp the blade is, you can need to pause, swirl, and blend every 30 seconds or so to ensure that it is evenly blended.
4. The mix should be thick enough to shape into balls at this stage. Squeeze between the fingers to see if this is accurate. It should not cling to your hands or break apart. However, it should remain intact. If it isn't holding together well, add some more coconut oil, then process once more. Re-blend with a little oatmeal or

unsweetened coconut if it's too moist. Shape 1 1/2 inch balls until all are prepared.

5. Place each ball on a plate or a parchment-lined baking sheet while you form them together (or you may use a baking mat of silicon). It can be placed on any flat surface.
6. The finely chopped coconut should then be placed on a different plate, cutting board, or another flat surface. It's best to use finely shredded, so it clings more. One by one, softly press each ball into the coconut until it adheres to all sides. Fill an airtight jar halfway with the mixture. Hold for up to a week in the refrigerator. A total of 22 balls are formed from this recipe.

45. CHICKEN BEETROOT AND BROCCOLI SALAD WITH AVOCADO PESTO

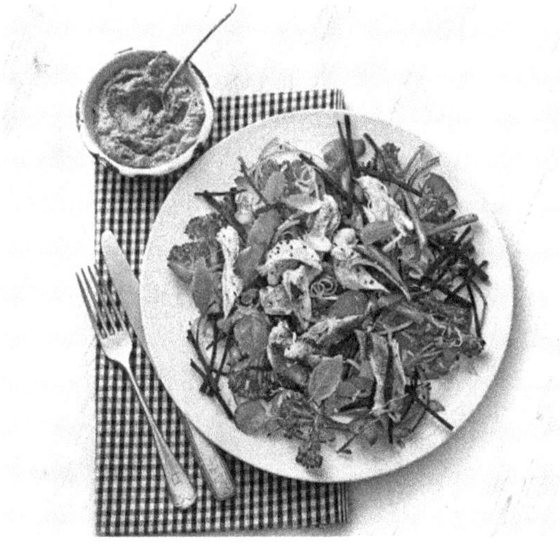

Serving: 4

Preparation time: 15 minutes

Nutritional values: Calories-320kcal|Carbs-8g|Protein-29g|Fat-18g

Ingredients

- 250g broccoli with thin stems
- 2 teaspoons rapeseed oil
- 3 breasts of chicken (skinless)
- 1 thinly sliced red onion
- 100-gram bag of watercress
- 2 stripped and cut into chunks or grated fresh beetroots (approximately 175g)
- Nigella seeds, 1 tsp.

For Avocado Pesto

- A small pack of basil
- A single avocado
- 1/2 crushed garlic cloves
- 25g walnut pieces, crumbled
- 1 lemon, juiced, and zested
- 1 tablespoon rapeseed oil

Directions

1. Take a large pot of water to a boil and steam the broccoli for 2 minutes. Drain and then rinse with cool water. Warm a griddle pan, mix the broccoli with 1/2 teaspoon rapeseed oil, and cook for 2-3 minutes, stirring once, until scorched. Leave to cool. Season the chicken and dust it with residual oil. Griddle for 3-4 minutes on either side or until done. Allow cooling before slicing or shredding into chunky bits.
2. Prepare the pesto next. Take a couple of basil leaves and put them aside to garnish the salad. Place the remainder in a food processor's little bowl. Scoop out the avocado flesh and mix it with garlic, oil, walnuts, 1 tablespoon lemon juice, 2-3 tablespoons cold water, and some spices in a food processor. Move to a small serving dish after mixing until smooth. Allow the residual lemon juice to sink into the sliced onions for a few minutes.
3. Arrange the watercress on a wide platter in a pile. Toss in the broccoli & onion, as well as the lemon juice in which they were soaked. Add the beetroot and chicken on top; just don't mix them together. Represent with the avocado pesto and a sprinkle of preserved basil leaves, lemon zest, and nigella seeds.

46. RED CHICORY PEAR AND HAZELNUT SALAD

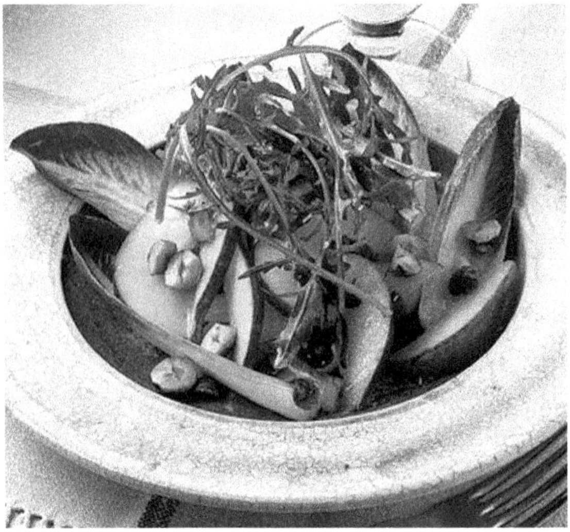

Serving: 4

Preparation time: 20 minutes

Nutritional values: Calories-176kcal|Carbs-8g|Protein-2g|Fat-15g

Ingredients

- 2 heads red chicory (or white chicory if red isn't available)
- 2 red, Williams's pears, fully ripe
- A big bunch of rocket leaves
- 25g toasted and diced hazelnuts
- To prepare the dressing
- Optional: 1 teaspoon green peppercorns (in brine)

- 2 tablespoons olive or hazelnut oil
- 2 tablespoons medium salad oil (sunflower or safflower)
- 1 teaspoon sherry vinegar or apple cider vinegar

Directions

1. **Prepare the seasoning.** If you're utilizing the green peppercorns, gently crush them with a wooden spoon in a bowl or in a mortar and pestle. Add the oils, then vinegar, and season with salt to taste.
2. Slice the chicory stalks off at the root and remove any limp or sore outer leaves. Carefully divide the leaves and place 5-6 on 4 plates, chopping or cutting every one into pieces if they are big.
3. Remove the pears' stalks and cut them in half lengthwise. Remove the cores and finely slicing the fruit. Place half of the dressing on each of the chicory leaves and place the pear slices on top. Season the rocket with salt and pepper and drizzle with the remaining dressing. Toss the leaves slightly and layer them on top of each salad. Serve with a sprinkling of almonds.

Conclusion

The Sirtfood Diet has become increasingly common in recent years, partly thanks to celebrities such as Adele's. It seems to have been trendy to be on a diet. Everyone wants to look elegant and modern, and they buy new clothes. We want to turn heads as we step into a room, but being on a diet will drain all of your strength without you getting anything out of it if the diet you're on isn't adequately controlled by a health practitioner or at least recommended by one expert.

The diet is dependent on a family of proteins in the body known as sirtuins, which regulate metabolism, inflammation, as well as other vital bodily functions. Sirtfoods, or foods recommended in the Sirtfood Diet, are rich in sirtuins activators that can help the body produce more sirtuins. The theory is that the more sirtuins our bodies have, the better they would be able to control metabolism, suppress inflammation, and so on.

"The diet focuses on eating a low-calorie diet rich in SIRTs (sirtuins), a family of proteins which have been shown to play a crucial role in keeping cells safe and can minimize inflammation and delay aging," according to the researchers. "It's believed that by consuming these foods, those genes that improve metabolism & burn fat would be activated."

The sirtfood diet is a better way to lose weight quickly without drastically reducing your junk food intake by triggering the same 'skinny genes' pathways by exercise and fasting. Certain foods include synthetic polyphenols, which place a gentle weight on the cells by activating genes associated with simulating the effects of fasting & exercise. The sirtuin pathways are activated by polyphenol-rich foods. An eating schedule rich in such sirtfoods encourages weight loss without losing muscle mass while still preserving overall fitness.

Integrate sound sirtfoods into your diet for good and embraced weight loss, booming energy, & inspiring well-being. Through this diet, you can boost weight loss and help combat a variety of illnesses by turning on the muscle versus fat absorbing forces. The sirtfood diet is an easy, well-proven method of weight loss. Flavorful, easy-to-make meals, as well as a maintenance schedule for deferred achievement. The sirtfood diet is a conscious, not restrictive, eating plan that is generally accessible and friendly. This is a diet plan that allows you to take your knife and fork and enjoy eating delicious, balanced food while still reaping the nutritional and weight-loss benefits.

CPSIA information can be obtained
at www.ICGtesting.com
Printed in the USA
BVHW081015070421
604341BV00006B/667

9 781914 358883